Schizophrenia and Anxiety

Mark Ellerby

chipmunkapublishing
the mental health publisher

Mark Ellerby

Published by
Chipmunkapublishing
United Kingdom

http://www.chipmunkapublishing.com

Copyright © Mark Ellerby

ISBN   978-1-78382-535-6

Introduction

Psychologists often quote case study examples of patients to illustrate to their readers and students the sorts of anxiety problems they work with. What follows is a first-hand experience of not only what these problems are like and also how the sorts of help which I have received enable them to be more bearable.

The problem of living with anxiety is much the same as the coping strategies in the text book approach which I hope the drama in this narrative compellingly brings to life. This is not a book on how to cope with anxiety so much as to try and get across to those who have never experienced it is what life with nervous problems are like.

The focus of much of this book then is on anxiety which in my case is caused by schizophrenia. As that illness is the cause of my anxieties this book is not called 'Essays on Anxiety.' That said many magazines on depression and schizophrenia will also publish articles solely on anxiety so what is in here may be useful to sufferers of these illnesses too.

So the hope still is that coping with these extreme anxiety problems may also help those with milder conditions and the thought that if schizophrenia can be overcome then many other anxiety related problems may also be tackled. Schizophrenia is definitely something to be anxious about. Of course a lot also depends on one's own courage so it is relevant that I do not count myself as a brave person.

What has happened in my case is that I have muddled through and gradually been exposed to sources of my anxiety and slowly learned to ignore it. From being too scared to leave my flat to being able to go out and about doing normal activity took a long time (two years) and what follows are my experiences in making that transition.

Anxiety can be a severe condition and so is often treated by a benzodiazepine such as diazepam or lorazepam, none of which have proved even minimally effective in my case. This book is also written for sufferers of anxiety who fall into this small group and for those who experience extreme anxiety for whatever reason or cause.

To begin then *suffering* from anxiety is the key term for this book. Anxiety, especially when it involves panic attacks, is a very disabling problem and can have a major impact on ones quality of life, and is some ways is like having a serious physical illness. I hope some impression of the severity of the condition comes through in this book.

In my case the experience of daily panic attacks has required a lot of support from the psychiatric system and in the form of living in supported accommodation. The helpful social contact this provides living with other people with a range of other conditions and diagnoses is also discussed in this book.

This experience and the benefits and problems this creates are also outlined. This aim here is to convey what this sort of living is like, not only to friends and relatives but also to people with anxiety disorders who might be considering this as a therapeutic option.

It may occur to some readers that all you need is courage or strength and the problems I will outline in this book will be solved by an act of will. That is not my experience however and for me there is a daily struggle to learn about and how to live with the problem. After a while you realise that you must each day as it comes.

It may be objected that if a person is so anxious how can they write a book about it? The answer is that some days are better than others and it is the intervening periods when I am relatively calmer that I begin to write. Although such writing is retrospective it is so close to the immediately experience of fear to be quite accurate.

One final point is that in writing this book it helped my battle with anxiety to refer back to what I have written previously to remind myself of what I have written in my other books entitled the stages of schizophrenia to remember other different coping strategies.

My experiences with anxiety

Anxiety then is a specific term the effects of which in my case are heightened by adrenalin rushes brought on by fear and mild levels of panic which creates a kind of palpitation effect in the body. Mostly though the focus for me is anxiety which manifests itself as nerves. The result of these nerves is a kind of paralysis of mind and body to which the only response is to wait until it wears off.

Taking lorazepam for me is a way of grasping at straws, a fact recognized by my psychiatrists. I am prescribed it even though it is both ineffective and addictive, though my levels of its consumption are closely monitored. The hope for me is rather that it has some kind of placebo effect though I doubt this.

Nothing in my life had prepared me for the anxiety I have had since leaving school. Prior to that I had exam nerves and interview nerves, the butterflies in the stomach on starting my first job but anxiety and fear are different. For one although your stomach churns with fear most of my nerves tend to be in my back and the backs of my arms rather like a pain that you simply cannot get rid of.

When I had anxiety at school, say when sitting my o-levels, this was accompanied by an adrenalin rush. I have heard it said however that there is good adrenalin and bad. In exams the nerves were accompanied by good adrenalin but with my current nerves there is both a more intense and unpleasant feeling of anxiety together with bad rushes of adrenalin – a much more potent combination.

People who complain of being 'bad with their nerves' are sometimes referred to 'anxiety management' classes by doctors. In my case I spent more time experimenting with everyday different ways of trying to cope and less with techniques like meditation, relaxation tapes or muscle exercises and the like (none of which I could understand enough to apply successfully). My CBT consultant also expressed some skepticism about this kind of approach to nerves.

So what do I do to stop being anxious? The most obvious adaption and the first to occur to me was simply to get up on a morning, sit in a comfortable chair and try to drink a cup of tea. This calms me down a little bit. This can be difficult as I often feel anxiety when I first wake up and the temptation is to simply stay in bed.

The reason for this is that it does require some effort and energy to get to the chair in the first place. This could appear as simply to try to avoid confronting ones problems but the experience to my mind is at least as indicative of the fact that it requires some strength to do this at all. It often takes me a couple of hours to do this. The reaction is not that because the anxiety often lasts the better part of the day it is better simply to stay asleep. It is not a decision that you take consciously as such it is just that it tends to reduce the anxious feelings when lying 'safely' in bed (perhaps in the feotus position) as well as the fact that you get up at a particular point when you feel strong enough.

After getting 'cleaned up' there can be a vulnerable moment when the lack of distractions of being in ones own room could make the mind wander onto the anxiety causing thoughts. It is necessary to find distraction by going visiting a neighbour for a chat which can be quite a lengthy affair. Indeed some such chats can in my experience last for up to five hours and even these are not totally effective!

Keeping busy is not high on my list of priorities for dealing with anxiety (I was later to change my mind about this). Some ways of doing this are ruled out because of the levels of concentration they require and for example I often find it difficult to read until after the anxiety wears off. More mundane things like cooking and cleaning are distracting to some extent but apart from the aesthetic pleasure of the end product (eg a tidy room) usually fails to make much of an impact on my nerves.

Keeping busy and being distracted are of course bound up together to some extent. Being a nervous person, as I sometimes refer to myself, I cannot watch or listen to violent movies, computer games or music – all things I used to enjoy before my nervous problems. Coming to terms with the window on the big bad world has always been a trigger to add more reasons for being nervous on top of those I already have.

The consequence is that what seem to be, at the level of common sense, the usual ways of coping with nerves are often very ineffective, if I could describe them as possible ways of coping at all. This has a further consequence for me in that there are less things to do 'around the house', the safest and most natural environment for me, and puts the emphasis on socializing and walking.

Going for a walk is then the next and one of the most effective strategies for me. It is best to have company and to go to somewhere isolated in my case. It is also necessary to choose the venue carefully. Again in my case I think woodland or rivers have the most successful calming effect but often foot public paths through fields and the like can also work just as well. Again I do not find this sort of therapy totally effective all the time though often it calms me down completely.

My meditation instructor advised me that if you do not remember anything at all about meditation remember this: control of breathing and taking deep breaths is the most important thing. I am very much aware that too long spent inside ones home with prolonged and high levels of anxiety does produce shorter more rapid breathing while being out and about during exercise on a walk forces the body to breathe more deeply.

Nevertheless sometimes this strategy works and sometimes it does not. At one point on a recent walk I started to get into the rhythm of my stride and focused a little more on the physical exercise than what was on my mind and causing the nerves. This enabled me to go through populated areas (rather isolated rural ones), which are normally an anxiety trigger, with relative ease. I was able to take my mind off my surroundings.

It has often occurred to me that there is no need to be afraid of being visibly anxious even in a crowd. Most people would I tell myself probably think that you are agoraphobic or some such and simply ignore you. This immediately recalls to my mind one such instance of panic breathing whilst in a department store and nobody seemed to bat an eyelid!

In fact crowds are in some ways easier to deal with than isolated footpaths because nobody specifically says hello to you in such environments. On a foot path you are individually acknowledged while in a crowd there is more anonymity. Buses are by far and away the most difficult because therein people cannot simply say hello and walk past you as on a footpath or in a crowd.

Instead you must sit as calmly as you can for the length of the journey – something I find difficult to do even for five minutes. The only good point about them compared to a foot path is that nobody says hello and looks at you directly unless of course they already know you. I always also find being amongst friends easier on my nerves than meeting or being around strangers.

On going anxiety beginning at the start of each day for a number of years (nearly four in my case) often produced the immediate response of staying or going back to sleep to avoid it. This rapidly becomes a habit to the point that it occurs even on well days as the body rapidly gets used to and requires more sleep. It is also a hard habit to break as such anxiety is itself very tiring, so reinforcing the sleep pattern.

Another consequence is that while on the sick with this problem is to find an enjoyable activity to keep the same level of energy and motivation in life. Otherwise it is easy to become so bored that the habit of going to sleep gets an even stronger hold on a person so that we sleep because there is nothing better to do. Again this can be a difficult habit to break.

Anxiety and the sleep response also create another curious and at times unpleasant outcome. Ones metabolism races as the heart rate speeds up while one lies still. In this respect there is rarely a calming response and it is often the case that once I get over the 'morning phase' as I call it my pulse rate eventually returns to normal, though not always.

It is also easy to 'give in to nerves' and I have often heard it said that 'you have to fight it.' Any prolonged anxiety is such a battle of the will but you have to proactive with it. So often before a walk or going into a supermarket (for example) I have to overcome the psychological barrier that I will be more anxious while being out and about.

Again another useful strategy is to 'keep your strength up' which requires eating and proper attention to diet and the like. Without this high levels of anxiety can soon make you dizzy and sometimes you just do not feel like eating or even expending the energy to make a meal. The microwave sometimes comes in handy for me at these moments.

Having creature comforts often helps me allay the causes of anxiety and give my flat a homely feel. To this end I expend much time and effort to this aspect of my life and the buying of such homely things often helps keep my spirits up. Nevertheless one cannot go on and on with this strategy.

Alcohol consumption is another tricky issue for dealing with anxiety. My CPN suggested 'a few drinks may help me.' Generally I tend to agree with this statement but even just a few drinks can act as a depressant and so sometimes this too is best avoided. There are warnings with anti-depressant or anti-psychotic medication to 'avoid alcohol' although many people I know with the mental health system take scant notice of this.

Some people I know like to relax with a drink late at night and helps with getting to sleep. However the best context for me is to drink socially, often while eating some pub food while sitting in the sun. At these times the relaxation effect of good food together with a group of friends and fine weather combines with the relaxation that comes with alcohol. This is also important to helping keeping you spirits up (of the non-alcohol variety!).

Another particular problem with high anxiety levels is that it makes concentration for driving very difficult, something which adds to the dangers of driving whilst on drowsiness causing medication. This makes life in general and getting away from it all in particular much more restrictive and I feel my ability to cope with this problem is thus very much impaired.

The next phase of anxiety

Anxiety too can be a deteriorating condition. I have had to abandon many of these strategies as it has become more difficult to leave my room. This has, however, necessitated the adoption another ways of trying to cope and new difficulties in doing so.

I think this has been a profound change in my problems and has lasted for about fifteen months so far. As a result I have put this phase into a new section.

The main problem is that confinement on ones own in a room means there is an initially lack of the usual strategies for dealing with anxiety. Being on ones own for a prolonged period intensifies the experience of anxiety and there is a lack of the usual distractions which I have outlined above.

This even gets to the point that the mind goes over and over the same problems and has no outlet. I would even go so far to say that it becomes obsessive. Gradually, once again, you learn to adapt.

The first strategy I have adopted is to try and play movies which and enjoyed before the illness. These usually hold good memories for me and do not require the concentration required by reading. Music and computer games are likewise useful.

But the more I do this and the longer this phase of the illness goes on I the more I find that the good memories wear off and I begin to associate the movie and its script with the experiences of anxiety. At the extreme the media simply becomes background noise and it may be just as well to simply leave a noisy fan on.

Something else is or becomes need instead or in addition to this. Again getting fifteen hours sleep each day on tablets is an occasional remedy but is not physically healthy. I often get back pain from doing this and variations in the period of artificially induced sleep can disrupt normal day to day living.

If one - for instance - sleeps thirteen hours during the night then after a few hours of being awake again it is not so easy to simply go back to sleep. Often you simply become drowsy for a few hours and then awake once more. This difficultly is more prevalent during two or three successive days of trying this strategy and so it is best reserved for the worst periods of anxiety and is usually effective only once or twice a week.

So once again I have started to try and devise alternative coping strategies. Taking a pride in ones personal space becomes even more important than before as, to reiterate, it is impossible to leave it and go out. This has got to the point that when I first wake up I do not make coffee or shower but vacuum up instead!

That may sound very unusual and is a little difficult to explain. The best I can explain is that like old movies I have always enjoyed this sort of thing and so the activity is therapeutic. As I said the anxiety I experience is often present from the moment I wake up and so something has to step in to distract me straight away.

Once again this cleaning up which I find helpful is not effective and does not take very long in any case and something else is required to immediately follow it. That usually means cleaning oneself up which is very refreshing and helps with my overall mood. I never feel so run down that I simply sit in a chair and slum it.

Then the daily question repeats itself: then what? I have managed to wean myself off my habitual twenty cups of coffee per day; though I think addictive would be a better word than habitual. Caffeine is no good for nerves even though it offers therapy in other respects. A glass of water sipped slowly is I find now just as therapeutic and very relaxing and for me, together with a relaxing bath, acquires new significance whilst confined to my own space.

Eating can still be very difficult however and I have found that I have lost much weight during this current phase of anxiety: as much as one stone in two months. This is often not detectable as the anti-psychotics often have the effect of weight gain. Mostly I eat fruit and perhaps the occasional sandwich which is just enough to get by on.

Sometimes the inevitable frustrations of confinement mean that such outlets are simply not enough and I feel an overwhelming desire to get out of my room. This has meant going outside the building of the project I live in simply in order to get fresh air. This is against my better judgment but is non-the-less necessary.

As in writing this essay I have often found it necessary to remind myself to do these things in case I forget one or two of them and in order to try and systematically combat the anxiety I have a list of them on my wall. My hope is that considered altogether in this way I can conquer the psychology that I can eventually conquer these problems and develop ever more effective routines for dealing with it.

Anxiety and isolation

After a sustained period of staying in – confinement would be a better word – you learn to adapt. This for me has been a very gradual process but during the past few weeks my months of confinement have now become slightly easier. It maybe that this outcome has been somewhat delayed in my case as it has always been normal for me to go out.

I have begun to compare my confinement to relatives in the village where I grew up who have had similar experiences due to premature bereavement of their partners and how they enjoyed the single life. I recall that various things acquired more significance in their life and have found that this has happened to me too.

When I have been so preoccupied with anxiety it is important to remember the little things in life which can help with relaxation. In my case I even forgot that anxiety creates muscle tension and that it does not take only a relaxing bath to counter this effect. I had to remember to massage parts of the body that a lack of walking and excess of sleeping can also contribute to.

In time you gradually forget what it is like to go all the time though initially I had to go through a phase of weaning myself off this. Time still passes very quickly even when there is no apparent activity and I rarely feel bored. I am so preoccupied with my fears and the voices which talk about them the clock still races round.

Something similar happens with respect to ones happiness. In order for anxiety to cause sadness or depression you have to notice the deterioration in ones life. You can be so caught up with fear that you rarely think about this. However whether the changes in ones life quality in the long term have this outcome I cannot yet describe.

You begin to appreciate the little thing more – like washing up – and even start to enjoy the more mundane aspects of life. I have found it necessary to replace one life style with another and so far this has not yet made me unhappy.

What comes to fill the time and the void that life like this creates is a highly individual thing: in my case I have started to develop and interest in computer games and music which were only casual pastimes for me before my anxiety. I have learned to rely on my own company and although difficult at first I now feel that I seek less distraction in socialising which had become a continual resource for a long period.

This raises an inevitable question in my mind: how will the staff at the mental health project I live react to this isolation? Since the idea of the project is that group living is a good way of providing emotional support how will this confinement be understood and tolerated? This has become an increasing source of worry over time.

Their first reaction must have been: where is Mark? It is so out of character for me that the change in my behaviour was immediately noticeable but instcad of coming knocking on my door they waited to see what would happen. After a short while they rang my CPN who once again was extremely worried about the change and his visits became more frequent, much to the relief of my family.

As time went on my contact with the staff became less frequent and this posed the following dilemma: would all this be seen as a sign of increasing illness or increasing self reliance? Strictly speaking a resident should be in frequent contact with staff – at least once a day – for the purposes of therapeutic input and medical observation.

But this requirement has become coloured recently due changes in the housing association and increasing office work. This has meant it has been easier to become isolated which if I had not learned to adapt so well could have had more serious consequences for my mental health.

That only leaves reading books on anxiety management but I am too anxious to do that either. There is one caveat to that some books on these matters where you can read a sentence, usually in the form of a maxim or concise statement, which you can discuss with a support worker.

It far easier to try and read and absorb books on anxiety by reading books comprising one sentence per page and then trying to understand (or apply it) but talking it over with a support worker. And there are such freely available in shops.

Watching Movies

I found a good way to relax was watching films thought most of the time I was not completely absorbed in it and unlike going shopping I was conscious of my anxieties at the back of my mind. The same was true of toying with the internet (my other major pass time).

Due to the decreased social contact at the project I live in watching movies acquired a new significance and I could go for two to three days particularly at the weekends without seeing anyone.

This also meant a reliance on phones calls from my family. Some days I waited all day for my mother to phone and afterwards I would feel better for a long time.

However when playing computer games with my friend Jamie I was able with the combination of activity and social contact to banish my anxious thoughts completely.

The benefit of these activities was chiefly because I was so completely absorbed in them I forgot I was there. Nevertheless it meant some escape from the fear. The more I try to keep busy the more escape I get. Being absorbed in a game the less my mind wanders onto my schizophrenic worries though the opposite situation is often true as well.

Hitting the Bottle

Being in the small group of people for whom benzodiazepines are not effective you are left to cope pretty much by yourself. There are other prescription drugs with an anxiety reducing effect and I have been prescribed a mood disorder drug called citalopram but I have not noticed much improvement there either. So what else?

To my knowledge that only leaves herbal remedies and aromatherapies which I have tried endlessly too and to no effect. The question now I have had to mask myself, given these severe and intolerant circumstances as I have described them in the essays about is what else can I do?

I think it is interesting to outline my experience with alcohol dependency with anxiety and how I have tried to keep it under control to some extent so far.

First things first here and that is exactly how much do you drink on a weekly basis. That is quite easy to answer: I get though about 40 bottles of Stella Artois and a Litre bottle or baileys in a week. Some people may laugh at this, especially 'heavy drinkers', but one thing leads to another...

With an alcohol problem you quickly learn that you something that has a bit of a kick. Some lagers with more than 5% volume of alcohol can do this but it is all too easy to start drinking spirits instead.

In my case for momentary panic attacks a shot of baileys does the trip but drinking Stella often has the same effect on me.

I am conscious that these sorts of descriptions are bordering on sounding like an alcoholic but so far I do not put myself in that category and so I currently regard them as something that goes with the territory of my anxiety problems.

Then there are other physical health problems involved which can be brought together at this stage. Excessive sleeping to avoid anxiety and excessive comfort eating leads to weight gain. These problems are compounded by my new and increasing reliance on alcohol and my equal inability to get out and about.

Nevertheless there is a need for support doing this and here my family and professional support can play a key role here too. When in my home village and staying at my parents overnight we can drive to isolated places and have a lengthy walk once or twice a week.

The best example of this is the twice yearly holiday on the Northumberland coastline which is un-crowded and for that matter unspoilt. The combination, after lengthy confinement in a room, of exercise, sea air and beautiful scenery is invigorating, therapeutic but above all relaxing.

This is supplemented by walks with my mental health support worker though here the route taking means we will pass other walkers which I find difficult. These restrictions lead back to a considering getting a treadmill – but now with a renewed urgency as I am over seventeen stone in weight.

One peculiarity with reliance on drink is that, as I have found, it is possible to go for fairly long periods without drinking and then, almost like a relapse, you are back to square one. I have found this to be true on a number of occasions and it seems to depend on variance with the level of anxiety I experience.

Equally curious is that when I am with my family I can get by with hardly any alcohol at all. Again that changes as soon as I get home. Then my nerves creep back into my mind and after a couple of hours successfully resisting the urge to drink I eventually give in. This is something that gets worse over time but it still leaves one to three days a week alcohol free however.

Eventually I came to the conclusion that the best strategy against drink as well as nerves is to be distracted. That can be achieved indoors but the most effective times are getting out and about with good company but that realisation as I shall now describe came about in different ways and with some resistance.

The worst thing about anxiety and its debilitating effects is that it destroys your life. You are simply unable to go about any normal activities including such things as work, leisure and education. Eventually for these reasons too it becomes clear that something had to be done.

Challenging the problem

This might seem an odd essay to follow on from hitting the bottle but it is from that condition that I have gone to get help. 'That condition' here encompasses both staying in my flat at the project I live in to avoid exposure to going out and drinking to calming my nerves.

I think having spent two years in my room was a very visible signal that this were getting much worse with my schizophrenia. Something had to be done. A meeting was called under the section 117 of the Mental Health Act and a risk assessment was to be done.

At the meeting where the staff from the project I lived in, my family, my Community Psychiatric Nurse and even my Psychiatrist. In my past experience sometimes in the psychiatric system having to apply mental law makes Social workers and the like feel a little uncomfortable about the coercion involved but not so here.

There was instead a definitive consensus that I should try and tackle these terrifying problems and I tried to resist every suggestion that they made. We talked for two hours and this ended by the conversation (I do not dare use the word argument) going around in circles.

Mainly I kept giving examples of times where I had actually tried already to get out and about and of the damage to my nerves this had done. I did want to repeat the experience and I kept reminded them that I had already had one nervous breakdown already which left me in a state of shock.

Nevertheless I was that tired from arguing about all this with a whole group of concerned helpers I caved in and agreed to go along with the help provided. I was in for a big surprise and have begun to make good progress which I shall now describe.

Paradoxically going out with a support worker took me a long time to get used to and initially used to raise my anxiety levels. It was not possible to go with her into a public place and so we began the process of trying to feel relaxed around her by but not going out at all. We began instead by her dropping in for coffee in the project I live in then by going for drives in her car.

Another factor here was that although the support worker was a very nice lady but after a year of shunning all social contact it took a long time to get used to a new person. The normal talking points when getting out and about didn't seem to make any impact on her but after a year of trying different talking points this got a little easier.

In the end I felt I better start talking about the bits of self help anxiety books I had bought and see if she could shed any light on the advise written there or on how to put it into practice. I think although she suggested some useful pointers on occasion to reiterate the main approach to try was overcoming the fear by *taking my mind off it*. This was also something the books mentioned.

My answer to that was to reiterate some situations caused me more of a problem than others. Then support worker had a good idea: why start this going out by visiting places I used to feel *comfortable* and *relaxed* in and then, step by step, begin to tackle more difficult places that I did not have the strength to cope with.

So I began to make a list of 'more difficult' and 'less difficult' although I could make a list of anything I found that could of gone under the heading of 'easy.' This was my list:

1 Hair dressers
2 Shopping Malls
3 Restaurants and Bars
4 Hotels
5 The staffs office in our mental health project.
6 City Centres
7 The Cinema
8 The Day Unit at our local hospital
9 The bus station
10 Getting on the bus

What makes one thing more difficult than others is the level of functionality and interaction with other people that is required while feeling afraid. As I mentioned earlier there is more capacity required in talking to people one to one as on a public footpath than there is in the anonymity of a crowd.

The least difficult was to sit in the drive at our local Macdonalds but I had to get used to the support worker I was assigned to first.

That happened both by being with my support worker in her car and travelling the 15 minutes into our local town and seeing 'strangers' through the window screens which to me act as a kind of psychological security barrier.

Once I got to MacDonolds she did the ordering, thankfully, but not knowing where to place myself, trying to look relaxed, and not to get involved with the cashier this proved very difficult and after six months of doing this I am still not used to or 'have mastered this.'

Once having got to MacDonalds the next step was to go and have another coffee in our local Further Education college. I have spent most of my life in one education establishment or another so this would hopefully bring back some good memories and be a familiar and relaxed environment to be in.

That proved to be true but it took a lot of effort to calm down even in this environment. My support worker and I sat in the car park watching the students coming and going and it took about ten minutes to get the courage to even get out of the car.

Walking towards the main entrance I felt highly visible and began wondering to myself whether I might lose my nerve. I kept talking to my support worker all the way to the cafe trying to distract myself in the conversation. I tend also tend to talk a lot when I am nervous. I am not sure how this actually worked but I did eventually calm down.

On one occasion however once I had got to New College I kept the conversation going for twenty minutes on an academic theme but once I stopped I suddenly became aware of my environment and started feeling nervous again. At that point I had to leave and I was aware that the real challenge was to feel relaxed without being distracted.

It took six months to keep trying with this gradual approach. During this time things did not gradually get better and neither did we go one to do anything else more difficult. Nevertheless there are a few twists in the tale so far.

The first is that once I have spent a couple of hours out with my support worker the rest of the day is much easier. Simply getting a look out of the project and the room I have spent two years in gives me a tremendous lift and puts me in a much more sociable mood with the people I live with.

Even though the rest of the day often becomes less anxious and seems much more therapeutic my nerves do not always go away completely and I still need to drink but those two hours out of the project enhance my ability to cope with immeasurably.

There is one major caveat to all this. The mornings are still a very anxious time. I rarely have the strength to get out of bed but one I get cleaned up and have breakfast (a vital daily ritual) and on those Tuesdays and Fridays when my support worker is due I usually go through the same old panic attacks and fears as I anticipate the challenges that lies ahead.

After a year of such support this still remained a significant obstacle and has not got any easier. This has the consequence that if the support worker was ever not there would I ever be able to go out by myself? Time will answer this one, I thought.

After a while however time did answer some of this: I actually began to look forward to my appointments with my social worker. The reason was that I felt more confident getting out and about with her and more talkative in her presence, though by this point the nerves still had not gone away.

After such a long absence from society I had to relearn my social skills. Some of this meant developing new skills and some remembering the skills I had and the conversations I had with my support worker have been instrumental here.

Then gradually she began to suggest ideas about coping on my own. This started with walk around the garden each day, unaccompanied, and then walking down the street. What follows is how I began to cope with more and more difficult venues.

Going shopping

So there is a further question about dealing with anxiety and that is sooner or later you are going to have to cope with it on your own. I have tried to be pro-active about this and been quite surprised by the results. I booked myself into a hotel over night, by myself, and talked to the receptionist and taxi driver and even went into a few local shops to boot. But what if it doesn't work?

The good thing here is that if you went into the hotel bar and felt it was too much of a strain all you have to do is go back to your room (though it is often necessary to bring your own DVD player to pass the time!) I never felt particularly natural doing this and to date walking around our local shopping mall with my family takes place in much the same circumstance – in that you can go back to the car if you need to – but it increases my confidence greatly.

Going to a shopping mall has ready-made conversation and I like discussing the pros and cons or buying different items. I am much more relaxed doing this with a family member though if I am left alone too long outside the shop my anxieties creep back into my mind. All this, and including the retail therapy, tends to keep me calm and might possibly help avoid depression.

So then the support worker suggested why don't we why not go into a shop rather than New College? Once again this seemed the logical next step and was something I was able to do with my family. To do this was still frightening but still seemed possible and valuable, even without my usual family help doing this sort of thing.

At one point my support worker wandered off to look at another display within the shop and I was left on my own. She suggested this to me before we went into the shop and it worked quite well at first as I was engrossed in looking at the products.

Although it was easy to go into Boots and browse for a while but after standing in the queue at the checkout I felt nervous the whole ten minutes (which seemed much longer). Nevertheless it was easier than passing the kiosk at MacDonalds but even so it was not possible to go in our local supermarket since I had past experiences of that.

Eventually you run out of new places to go and this means keeping trying with those places which you have least nervous associations. That adds to the degree of anxiety but these problems are merely the same as getting out of your room in the first place and so can be overcome despite the perception of apparent difficulty.

It is necessary to get out and about every day for some therapy. The difficulty of this problem is that it is not easy for family and support workers to give one person so much time and input. The hope is you gradually come to do this yourself but without intensive (ie daily) help getting to that point (judged by my current rate of progress) can take a number of years.

Graded exposure again is the key and it is necessary to start with situations you feel comfortable in and which have some degree of familiarity and then introduce others including ones which have bad memories of anxiety.

The CPN described the goal of his support role is that social inclusion and really that is the best name for it. Anxiety not only prevents doing every day things but from meeting new people and I find it hard to talk and interact with new residents at the project I live in, or strangers, as I sometimes call other people outside the project.

Certain routine activities, like going to the supermarket, become very difficult with high anxiety levels but some are unavoidable. Having a haircut is one. To solve this it is necessary to park outside the salon and go at a time like a Wednesday afternoon when there are very few other customers.

The possibility of distracting conversation at such times is very strained. There are the inevitable questions such as 'what do you do?' or 'are you going out tonight?' I find it easier to invent answers here than say I have an anxiety disorder. I find it hard to start conversation about other topics.

All the same such appointments only last twenty minutes and they can seem fairly arduous. I dread the experience before it actually happens but afterwards it is again not as bad as it seems.

Making progress is not a linear thing: there can be set backs and sometimes very serious ones. These occur because you are always pushing the boundaries of your comfort zones and trying to so means you can try and take on too much.

One example, already noted, was trying to watch the cinema at our local shopping Mall. Going shopping is an achievable aim most of the time as is going to the Malls restaurants to eat. But sitting in a cinema instead of being distracted by the movie has instead on occasion been a disaster for my nerves.

The beguiling thing here is that this did not seem any different than sitting in a restaurant. But once having been to a Mall and a restaurant and having coped ok with both I tried to go into a cinema and panicked. I lasted 20 minutes and had to leave.

The problem is that if I felt that 9/11 started to occupy my mind and that I was in a lot of danger. It reminded of the reason I stopped going out in the first place that doing so I was in a lot of danger and that the risks were too great and simply unacceptable.

My initial panic reaction subsided after a short time but I was left with the feeling that I wouldn't be going back there in a hurry. Eventually I calmed down completely but the experience of cinemas left a lasting impression on me mainly it is so easy for the mind to go back to thinking about being anxious and triggering off a bout of nerves.

 One final point is that being able to do something like going into a shop to buy something is not the goal of social inclusion. Rather it is to be able to function normally *without anxiety.* That is much more valuable and much more difficult. The lesson here is not to give in.

Family Help

I often find it much more therapeutic to be at home than the project I live in and indeed often feel the loss of not being there.

During these visits I do not feel the need to drink or eat excessively and enjoy distractions such as playing *trivial pursuit.*

That changes when I get home again and even after twenty minutes or so and I as also mentioned above fall back into the same habit of eating and drinking alcohol.

It is surprisingly still better to get out and about with ones parents than sitting around at home. This in our case often involves going to shopping malls and places to eat.

Living with my family alas is not possible and so the next best support comes from the sheltered housing project I live in.

There are even times when I start yearning to go home because living in the project simply makes no impact on my nerves at all.

It is often commented to me by family that I always less anxious when I am at home, occupied with something. This usually means some form of activity such as playing with my nephew, talking to my parents over a few drinks, or writing this book etc.

Looking at it from this perspective the problems I have while at the project seem to arise because there is less going on. The only solution then appears to be looking at books on anxiety management to find new ways to cope - once again - when in isolation.

At this point a new and surprising difficulty began to present itself: it is possible to be very dependent on one's family for this kind of help. Almost like a kind of institutionalisation it is necessary to wean oneself off this kind of support and cope on one's own.

In fact the situation is very like the stereotypical image of kids who have had a sheltered upbringing and then who have to cope all of a sudden in the 'big bad world', though I think the situation of having continual panic attacks may well be more difficult.

My own upbringing was sheltered as by definition was my ten year stay in sheltered accommodation and I think this has affected my ability to cope around new and strange situations but since my more recent anxiety problems this sort of problem has become more pronounced.

However just like having to confront any anxiety causing problem the situation is always that you have to face it eventually without the help.

At this point my support worker tried to encourage doing things on my own, starting by having a walk in the garden and followed by a walk down the street.

Looking back the key for me has been as much about self help as it has about having support. Friends and family can only listen for so long about anxiety. Each time they pick up the phone and ask how have you been today I always say another anxious day and leave it as that. They have problems of their own to contend with and must switch off emotionally to the extra burden of my anxiety problems.

Thankfully conversation need not always focus on this and it often helps me to talk about other people than it does to offload my own problems. This is also a good reason to live in Sheltered Accommodation as help dealing with it is a professional job not a families responsibility though even with this kind of help there are limits to how much support is available.

Sheltered Accommodation

There are times while living in sheltered accommodation, when there are few people around to talk to, so that I miss being at home. This can be a prolonged feeling lasting up three or four days.

During these times I am partially distracted by using the internet and listening to music as I have mentioned above. The problem is that these activities are nowhere near as distracting when compared to doing the same things at home or, for that matter getting out and about.

Normally though there are significant intervals when there is a lot of therapeutic social contact with long standing friends and this provides an opportunity to 'catch up.'

Although not as good as being at home the support I receive is generally very good and keeps me functioning at quite a high level (as for example being to write this book).

It also complements the other kinds of support I receive from family, holidays, sheltered housing staff, CPNs and psychiatrists and with the exception of family it is hard to know which is the most effective.

Listening to other people's problems is a good distraction to avoid dwelling on one's own which has been the key problem dealing with the anxiety during the year long isolation which I have experienced and described above.

The sad side of all this is that you can come to depend on this social contact to enable you to cope and in my experience if anyone is cured, transferred or as in one tragic case in our project dies such support is reduced.

The remaining the social side of our group living consists in dropping in on the other residents for a chat and cup of coffee and keeping all our doors open to be reminded of each other's presence. All this creates a very therapeutic atmosphere but it is limited by the fact that it is not 24/7.

Often the people I live with will sleep through the day, go home for the weekend or out on the town three days a week, as each tries to overcome the feeling of boredom of having little else to do. At present there is no social scene as and when you want it which up until now has always been one of the major pluses of group living.

The death of our mutual friend Fred who was often around and available whenever you felt like dropping in for a chat changed that for good and is a salutary reminder of how good group living can be and what its limits are too.

Having being on a hospital ward there was a constant turnover of new faces and this has also been true of the staff and residents in the project I live. Over the years however (ten in fact) I have gradually began to stick to people I know and shy away from new social contact. This has significantly reduced the therapeutic side of collectively living and fred is a prime example.

What happens is that you can quickly lose your social skills after, as in my case, after a year of isolation and that the thought of trying to reacquire them does itself become a source of anxiety. Being slow to adapt to meeting new people (staff and residents) is the main problem and it seems this can only be done by trying to strike up new conversations or by finding some common interest.

So the problem of anxiety in the morning presents itself here in another way: without the proper social contact it takes a long time for the panic and fear to wear off. This difficulty was exacerbated by a lack of opportunity for staff contact. In our project there is one member of staff for ten residents so that puts the emphasis on self reliance and group contact.

It was for this reason that the service manager suggested that one of the staff could make an intervention in the morning time, shortly after I awoke, to try and solve this problem. They could only spare fifteen minutes but hope is that a short chat may have the same effect as the lengthier outings with my support worker and relax me for the rest of the day.

The main difficulty here is that if were to push this point too much they (the staff at our project – might decide that I need a higher level of support and transfer me some were else. My reaction to that would be to keep quiet as it has taken a decade to get to homely feel of where I live now and to grow the relations that have now become established.

Bar Meals

After a while I decided – without prompting – to try and get out and about with a friend instead of the support services. I opted to go to a local pub and have a bar meal with a friend. Not knowing how this might turn out I was surprised how relaxed as I was and by the fact I managed to sit in the pub for over two hours!

Food is a great relaxation therapy! This is not just down to taste and quality. Food, in fact, has a big impact on your mood and brain chemistry and I have found a good diet is necessary to combat severe nerves. My local day centre provides expert advice on diet and it is easy to overlook essential constituents which may help such problems.

It may be objected how can you eat if you are so nervous? The answer to this is that being sufficiently distracted and so able to relax appetite has not being a problem. Indeed the fact is good food and some alcohol in a social context heightens the feeling of relaxation immeasurably.

This often applies while eating at home and I spend a lot of time thinking about meal times, given that on some days there is little else to do. Some days revolve around meal times and it has also helped my quality of life to eat the finer things in addition to having a glass of wine or lager.

Afterwards I began to wonder why this seemed easier to accomplish than with a support worker and found what I should of realised beforehand: namely that when I am out and about and engrossed in conversation I do not feel so aware of my surroundings. Because I was with a friend who I had known for ten years there was much more to talk about than with the support worker who had I known for only one year.

After that there was an immediate feeling of success, though it might sound curious to some that this feeling was not that of elation or of freedom and release from confinement. Why this should be I don't know but it did produce a feeling of optimism that after having done it once I could do it again. Once back at the project we even began to plan another excursion for the following week.

Looking ahead once again I began to wonder where else to go to take this next step. The temptation initially was to go somewhere quiet so as not to have a room filled with strangers but it also seemed logical to go somewhere busy to be more anonymous. In the end I opted to try the busier venue without really knowing if it would succeed but as with all such progress there is an inevitable element of risk. In the end you must confront the object of your anxieties to overcome them.

Hotels

After a while I began to have another idea: using the incremental approach why not look at staying in hotels further afield? To begin with it was possible to stay in hotels close to what has always been home then when it becomes possible to travel by bus or train (things which have featured high in my list of difficulty above) to go to new and interesting places further afield.

This venture has the interesting consequence for me that travel has a kind of carrot attached that I have always been interested in tourism and geography; it provided something of a distracting goal worth pursuing and an incentive to try it, despite the risks. Nevertheless the prospect at first did seem quite daunting and it seemed to me that the allure of the goal tempted me to give it a try despite however it might turn out.

Goal is the key word here: confronting anxiety and being able to do normal things is one goal but another concerns what I want to do in life is quite another. It reminds me not just about being able to function but that I can do things to improve my quality of life even perhaps to the point of being happy with it. This is a very important distinction to make and once the difference is realised – and it took some time for me to do this - it provides for a much more powerful source of motivation (most of the time anyway).

I think one of the reasons it took me awhile to do this was because I was concentrating too much on the sources of happiness before my difficulties and too little on what else life has to offer. Going on holiday with my family and to hotels have always been sources of therapy but it began to occur to me that seems to be something common to my age group and also that I would like to do it a lot more often.

Then a problem presented itself: the best time to go to hotels was to get out of the project since staying in my room concentrated my mind on the various anxieties. On occasion these nerves could last up to two days after which I would sustained some psychological damage. It is at these times that I most need to leave the project but the problem then became how would I have the strength to do it?

One answer I told myself was to have a holdall ready to go and do it at the drop of a hat. I was used to travelling with our local taxi firm and could make the reservation over the internet and stay in my hotel room if I was too nervous to go out. Nevertheless despite all of this sound reasoning I still did not have the strength required.

This proved to be a temporary problem and coincided with the work I was doing with my support worker: after a while she began to suggest why not try doing the first leg of a walk unaccompanied and meeting up after the first few hundred yards?

I readily agreed to this and did so because I recalled that in the past I needed a bit of a push to confront my fears, such as walking past our local shop, and things did not turn out so bad. Things however did not go so well the first time, almost to the point I felt I had taken a step back in terms of the therapy's progress. Nevertheless it did not put me off trying it again the week after.

Soon afterwards I began to see ways of combining these different strategies and decided to stay in a hotel near the village I grew up in. I knew of a few lovely relaxing places to go walking nearby and so was able to practice getting out and about by myself as well as having to leave the project and room and spend the night somewhere else.

This has the added bonus that I would be in a familiar environment (where I grew up) and hopefully would be not so nervous there. I might even manage a walk through the village, or so I thought, but otherwise could do almost as well sticking to outlining roads and paths.

Sometimes however even the best laid plans of mice and men go wrong and the hotel stay turned out to be another set-back. Rather than going walking I did not leave my room though the change of scenery was calming I was nervous around the hotel staff. It occurred to me not to go back there but did not dissuade me to try another hotel elsewhere.

After that I thought about the whole exposure to anxiety approach and it made me question again was I trying to do too much? Yet without another push from my support worker there would be no progress at all. What struck me about the results of the push was how quickly I bounced back and regain some optimism about the whole enterprise. It seemed that this sort of stop go progress characterised even when things seem to be improving a lot.

The turning point?

One day while out with a support worker and after a typically nervous morning things seem to get better all of a sudden. We went to get some stuff from Boots and it struck me why not look in NEXT? After that I wandered further round the retail park until I got to the supermarket. This was very high in my list of priorities but almost without thinking I went in again without any distracting supportive conversation.

My support worker went to the toilet and I was left alone to browse the movies and computer games. After about five minutes she came back. It did not seem like an eternity and we even stayed for another five minutes looking at the same products. Then we went back to the car, relaxing while we walked.

The curious thing was that *now* it didn't take a further push from my support worker to do this and I wasn't pushing myself. It just happened anyway and it was no big deal. There was no feeling of having achieved a goal or of making progress. Afterwards however I wondered could it be done again the same way?

Another curiosity was that I didn't start to analyse: was this a trend or a blip? I didn't worry whether it would be the same the next time we tried it. Indeed I could see a future when all such considerations would be in the past and perhaps I would never look back?

Then at one point at home the same old anxieties began to creep back into my mind and I began to be fearful about going out again. At this point I decided to go and see a friend at project I live in. At the time this was not possible so I kept busy while my family arrived.

This worked and I began to hope the rest of the day would reinforce the progress of my outing with the support worker. Even if it did not then least it was a start, I thought?

Even as things seemed to be improving new problems began to present themselves: my support worker suggestion of walking out into the garden by myself proved to me just how dependent I was on having the help of support worker and the project staff of the shelter I lived in.

This dependency was a kind of institutionalisation and it became apparent that it too must be challenged in much the same way as my symptoms of anxiety. I began to wonder how long it would take to tackle these new secondary problems and how difficult it would be.

So far so good

As I have stressed before in these essays one thing leads to another and because of the similarities in the nerve inducing situations listed from one to ten above. This is all the more remarkable because even at the upper end and most difficult place in my list this is still true. Namely when sat in a pub and being served a meal where there was other customers I managed to have the strength to sit among them for half an hour which is more than my local bus takes to the city centre.

The key however was – and it took me a long time to realise this – that being in such close confines to other people for so long was equivalent to sitting on a bus with other people for the length of the journey. The only difference was that being on the bus means you cannot simply get off if you feel too frightened but sitting in the pub made me feel like giving it the try.

Another idea occurred to me then: if you can try a lot of arduous challenges and handle each one individually and successfully why not try and combine them. It also became apparent at this point that progress back to normal functionality was to be sudden – like someone waved a magic wand – when compared to the slow but sure progress up to that point. It was scarcely to be believed.

Although I stopped trying to psych myself up it was still necessary at this stage to travel by car and go to Mac Donalds for a coffee while sitting in the car park for 15 minutes outside the first shop we were to go into. That is a seeming paradox which I have found difficult to explain but my support worker assured me it made sense!

Although there was some fluctuation we pressed on to the next goal which planning what to do when out and about by oneself. Going to the cinema and walking were the two most likely eventualities. Having been through a period of isolation during which I tried to rekindle interests I had pursued in the past I realised that it was the people rather than the activity which had made them enjoyable and that this made it impossible to go back.

So I began to think ahead instead. Following the social context of activity going for walks seemed boring and more arduous alone but it then occurred to me that once the endorphins were released the isolation would not matter so much. It took some time for me to realise this however.

The other main goal of going to this cinema cured a similar problem. Once able to get on a bus the immediate question is where you were going to go? Being fed up with shopping it took me a long time to realise that there were other distractions that could be done in isolation on a regular basis.

Then it hit me: why not just go out in order to relax? That was a more valuable goal than being dependent on some form of activity because there was nothing suitable to do once when out and about. This then became my new gaol.

So I thought a trip to the shops everyday might just give me a much needed lift. However it soon became apparent that spending three hours sitting by the river was quite boring and that such long visits had limited therapeutic value. On one such occasion I simply gave up and went home

As things progressed my perceptions began to change: being on a bus journey did not scem that it took an eternity but was in fact just 15 minutes long. Eventually when listening to a walkman the same journey seemed to take a mere 5 minutes.

On Holiday

I decided to go on holiday with a friend for a week. My initial impression was that this would be much more challenging than the simple overnight stay hotel described above. We never did the day trip to York before hand and in this sense too it was a big step rather than a gradual one.

Nevertheless I was not sure whether it would turn out badly or not. I kept having mental flashes about the challenge of being of being up there alone and doubts were also flashing to my mind during a severe terror attack was the thought that I would not cope so far from home.

The next day these doubts returned to being subconscious and I lost the immediate sense of the fear so that I nearly forgot them altogether. I decided to press on with the holiday and hoped the doubts would not resurface again.

All the same I tried to reason the whole thing through. I reminded myself that going for walks on the isolated familiar beach at Bamburgh castle was something I had done before and without incident. There were pubs and restaurants at Seahouses and these were not comparatively different from local pubs in Durham.

At this point I stopped comparing thinking that the exercise was somewhat fruitless. Instead I decided simply to go ahead and go on holiday without too much analysis.

Nevertheless it was necessary to go self catering to avoid hotel staff and to find somewhere secluded. My step dad drove the taxi (his part time job) and collected the key to the cottage as I found this quite frightening.

Good times and bad times

Very soon the outings got longer and longer without any increase in anxiety. At times this felt like striking out. I began to consider the possibility of outings by myself and even found that it was necessary to push myself to do this instead of conforming to a misplaced sense of obligation to the demands of family and social workers etc.

Another change here was I began to opt for exposure to the most frightening environments instead of easier ones. It is too easy to choose the soft option but in the end I began not to do so. It also became easier and quicker to bounce back after set backs.

During periods of milder anxiety my hope was to try the bach flower remedies together with the aromatherapy treatments including lavender. As I mentioned above these made no impact on my anxiety even though the rockrose was prescribed for terror...

My thought was and this may be true for some people at lower levels of anxiety the treatment would be effective lengthening the duration of time in between symptoms and it maybe that during ill phases you could say to yourself that the anxiety would wear off and I can get back not just to normal but happy intervals as well.

Following this line of thought it is necessary to pamper yourself as much as possible with retail therapy and getting out and about or whatever else works for the person concerned.

Now while all this seems very like common sense the acute nature of the problem prevents me in my case at least me thinking about this in this sort of way. However I think that subconsciously I am somehow kept going by doing this the advice is not completely unfounded and perhaps I have also avoided becoming depressed by it in this way.

It kept me going by making the most of the good times even including drinking alcohol but more especially by lots of family contact, also including baby sitting my niece and nephew. All of this gave me a definite lift.

Panic Attacks

One thing that stands apart in the experience of anxiety in terms of its severity is a panic attack. Once during the third week of attending a confidence class at my local day centre I had a panic attack in the class room but being so relaxed with the set up it did not force me to leave the class. The teacher gave me some lavender to inhale on a tissue.

After that I had another panic attack the next week in a local pub. I had bought some lavender and carried it around with me. To my great surprise I managed to stay in the pub and even get on a crowded bus.

Having being enlightened by the experience in the confidence class I was less inhibited by my surroundings and was not worried about what others would think. That would have heightened the anxiety but the lavender would have cured that too. There was no panic about panicking and I survived the whole experience.

Still the bus service seemed to take ages but I hung on in there to the very end. Once I got back home the familiar surroundings calmed me down and I had time to reflect: if it happened again I was willing to run the risk of panicking while out and about even if very far from home. Panic attacks are nothing to panic about, I thought.

Yet at other times during my frequent panic attacks I kept telling myself that this is the end, that I won't cope and my life would end. It was true that this was as severe and as serious as the terror could get. I was so scared that I never even began think about what I was experiencing and questioning the associated thoughts.

What did feature uppermost in my consciousness was the sensation of the adrenalin and the worry that I would be driven deeper into shock. Would I have another breakdown? Would I be able to recover from this? It is also true that you can panic about panic.

I tried to observe myself in this state of panic and notice what was happening. The easiest thing to notice was the adrenalin localised in my blood veins and this most frequently occurred in the calf muscles of my legs.

I tried to maintain a sense of detachment or critical distance on what was happening perhaps to try to rationalise it and persuade myself to calm down. This took a long time and didn't initially seem to work as a coping strategy.

I kept trying to tell myself there is no reason to panic or else to simply ride it out. Maybe I could watch myself in this state and realise that it would not get any worse or try to hold on until the symptoms went.

Uppermost in my mind was the question how long would it go on for. It seemed to some extent that it might be prolonged but actually went a lot sooner that it seemed it might. Before I knew it was all over and gain this gave me some confidence that if the panic recurred it could be dealt with.

The cognitive therapist

Eventually I was referred to a cognitive therapist at my local mental health day unit. I said I had tried to study books unsuccessfully on anxiety management and he said that particular part of CBT no longer focused on this because it did not work (this was something of a surprise to me because that is what my CPN referred me for). Instead we identified other problems I could be helped with including coming out of shock by using breathing exercises and also by increasing self awareness.

I was visibly nervous at our first meeting and his initial question for the next section was to account for this anxiety. Fear he explained was an immediate response whilst anxiety was different in severity and more prolonged. Looking like my anxiety might be the result of Schizophrenia he first wanted to know what my exact thoughts were step by step and why they caused me such anxiety.

I replied that meeting new people put me on edge and that at that point the meeting began to feel a bit like a job interview. The other main problem was the day unit itself and the numerous episodes of nerves which over a lengthy period resulted in a feeling of anxiety every time I had to attend there. As the interviews nerves faded it was the longer standing problems he wanted to concentrate on.

I was given the task of writing up what caused the nervous reaction, why my mind used to race when I felt so nervous and to reflect that there was no real need to be frightened. This was reinforced by talking it over with the help and the reassurances that there no real need to be anxious. Gradually though the conversation changed from the psychoses to focus on the nerves.

So I set about this task promptly. It occurred to me that because I had strong memories of anxiety and panic attending the day unit itself was it had lodged a kind impression in my mind that was difficult to dispel. This made it easier to remember and as usual the thought of going there was itself frightening but it was not an insurmountable difficulty.

Again I think this was because I was accompanied by a CPN in his car for fifteen minutes which was relaxing. Without that the general idea of the difficulties of going to the day unit would have been much more fixed in my mind.

After that the next obstacle is passing strangers in the hospital car park and after that sitting with other people in the hospital waiting room. That can up to ten minutes and if it was not for my coping strategies would seem a lot longer.

These strategies involved a mix of distraction and avoidance. On the distraction side I find listening to music on my mp3 player useful and on the avoidance side I like to wait outside the doctor's door (and not in the waiting room) and even to put my fingers in my ears (feigning hearing voices). I also had to leave by the emergency exit.

Another adaptive approach here was to befriend the staff and patients at my local day unit but this was genuinely ineffective until I passed the fear threshold and began to relax by talking to them rather than simply being in their company. That usually gave me a bit of a lift and helped make more manageable being in the waiting room. The problem remained however that each successive appointment at the unit followed the same pattern and also needed overcoming the anxiety anew.

After that account I was several given questionnaires about anxiety. They rated its severity and divided up into the level of anxiety giving equal weight to psycho and somatic effects. I didn't think the questionnaire reflected the severity of my problems as when the results were totalled up it came out that I was categorised as having only moderate anxiety...

There were the questions I scored highly on and others I did not. I wonder if I filled the form out right as it seemed my bodily reactions to the anxiety were not as severe as the levels of fear I experienced, except perhaps the levels of adrenalin and muscle tension. I didn't score highly on dizziness and several other key indicators.

After a while another task showed the anxiety up rather better. I had to rate my anxiety by severity and duration. I recorded it every hour of every day for two and a half weeks. I recorded about 17 hours of absolute terror and 16 hours of anxiety every six days. Occasionally this went on for six hours at a time and these were clearly the worst periods at other times it only lasted for an hour or two. Clearly then I had good days and bad which wasn't evident to me until I had done the recording.

After a further period of recording I noticed another difference. Whereas the worst periods tended to be in the morning and before going out and about this pattern began to change too. It became more random. I stopped dreaming of my schizophrenic worries (mostly about being responsible about 9/11) and thankfully the daily routine of lying in bed with my metabolism racing began to end.

I eventually lost some of my fears on having to out and about with my support worker and again this took a long time but I think it is at this exposure to doing so which has been the biggest help. She thought in contrast that it was due to number of reasons including the CBT and proper compliance with taking the anti-psychotic medication.

The CBT specialist tried for a long time to get controlled exposure to these sorts of triggers. I had to watch videos about 9/11 and to try to coexist with the fear, something which helped by having a support worker there at the same time but also by having to do this by myself as well. He asked a lot more questions about how it was triggered and I replied not just dreams but also flashbacks and noticing my subconscious awareness of it from time to time. Again this confirmed his graded exposure approach.

Deep regular breathing was recommended. I had read this often but never really understood how to do it until it was demonstrated. I felt like I might pass out the effect was so overwhelming. After twenty years of being in shock it was fantastic to get back to normal with this. I was told to practice this twice per day which proved quite difficult.

The pop psychological stuff seemed to me to be harder to master than physiological exercises like breathing and muscle exercises. Yet odd as it may sound I found it difficult to settle long enough to practice what I read or what I had learned in the CBT session. I decided in the end to rely on relaxation exercises as it is something that is difficult for me to do by oneself.

The CBT specialist even recorded a CD for me to listen to. Being paranoid about any pre-recorded media with my schizophrenia I found commercially available tapes were not things I could listen to at this time. But trusting my consultant I was able to get around this problem and I thought he did an excellent job of doing it. After that I started to try to follow his clear instructions much easier than books on anxiety management.

All these strategies that were being brought into play complimented rather than constituted the cognitive approach. I explained to the therapist that I felt people could read my minds and this was causing the anxiety. He was very interested in this and came up with ways of trying to question it.

One interesting strategy he confronted me with was would the evidence that people were really reading my mind count as a proof in it was actually happening. Say that any form of scientific or philosophical theory had to be 'proved' empirically to count as knowledge. He asked me could my belief this was happening be proved in the same way. Having been to university this sort of thinking resonated heavily with me and I did have a few doubts at that point that I might be being delusional.

On reflection I was initially a bit shocked by the cleverness of this suggestion and of the interesting initial strategy of the question but then I got to thinking about it more. The interpretation seemed to fit the facts and so it seemed scientifically verifiable.

Then the therapist suggested asking people in my feared places if they could actually read my mind. What did I think they would say? To this I responded that I would have thought they would not tell me the truth that they were actually doing this. This silenced the therapist as one of the things it seems to be the case with schizophrenia is that it accounts for almost everything that might be used to prove such beliefs delusional.

Not to be put off by all this however the cognitive therapist came up with another ingenious suggestion. Write a list of things to keep in mind and see if someone I could trust could guess what I was thinking.

The list comprised a variety of everyday things and places chosen by myself such as the name of a planet, a plant, an animal, a country, a song and so forth. The doctor let me choose what to list and said the range of items was scientific.

I had to do this test with at least five different people including friends, family and support workers. These were people I thought would not lie to me about reading my mind.

So I did the test and found no one could get the right answers and more than this I could see that the one question a friend did get right (the name of the planet mars) could as well have been coincidence because there were only nine planets from which to select.

Still I had the belief that my mind was sometimes being read by people so the therapist came up with another exercise. Every time I had this feeling I had to fill a form out about exactly what was happening.

The form included what I thought was being said and whether there might be some other explanation involved such as they might have been discussing something else entirely.

I was to keep making entries to the form every time these beliefs surfaced and to do this for an extended period of time, namely at least six months.

Looking back at the entries on the form I could visualise the situations that brought the belief in mind reading out and what the alternative explanation could have been at that instance. The collection of many such instances would it was hoped undermine the general picture of what was happening.

That general picture had taken a long time to crystallise and would take a lot of form filling to undo this but after a period of time it became obvious this was not working.

The CBT consultant also asked me why don't you just ring the CIA and see if they are are looking for you? To this I replied I wouldn't take the risk so he said why dont you ask the people who are reading your minds if they are going to report you. To this I said I didnt think they would tell me the truth. It seemed that every way he posed the problem the delusions came up with an answer.

One consultant I had virtually frog marched me up the street to somewhere I was frightened of instead of getting into an analysis about it. He saw my look of fear and being threatened he seemed to agree that the problem was real enough and didnt make any suggestions about what to do.

The CBT consultation lasted for a total of 18 months but finally came to an end where I think he had done all he could. Interestingly I was left with the impression there was only so much insight that a therapist can build on even when it is there to work with.. The work with the support worker went on however and again I think things made a little more progress with this two.

Rebuilding Self-confidence

Once I learned the relaxation techniques the next task was to rebuild my self confidence as my nerves had had a shattering impact on this.

I was referred to a confidence building class at my local day centre, as the relax class was full. Going there was easier because I went with a friend from the project I live in. It was also easier finding a class to do the CBT training in instead of trying to practice it at home.

The first thing that struck me was I knew some of the other people who had signed up to the same thing – people I would never have assumed would have had a problem with confidence. Perhaps we can exist behind some convincing facades. I asked my support worker about this and she assured me it was so.

The class began with each of us stating what we experience in terms of lack of confidence and what we hoped to get from doing the class. Thinking about this I realised I said that I was Ok talking about subject I knew about – including mental health but also computer games and others – but found it very difficult to talk about anything else.

This was also a great way of breaking the ice and after listening to other peoples problems allowed me to get to know them very quickly. Up until that point I stuck to the people at the day centre who I had known for a long time and it was a immediate confidence boost finding I could meet new ones. The hope for me to be able to talk to other strangers – in a bar for example.

The said benefits were much more numerous including energy, assertiveness, increased self respect and so on. Lots of pop psychology books promised this and more. It did occur to me that this amounted to a rather rosy picture of what life was going to be afterwards.

Building confidence is often not something that can be done overnight and I was surprised to find the course lasted one hour each week for the full academic term (ten weeks). After that I realised the process was a very gradual one.

There was also some homework to be done which required some thinking about and again this required some effort. It said that assertiveness was an attitude and looking this up I found the definition to be a mental position. I began likening it to other attitudes like. When I asked about this it was better to see it as a behaviour.

I think I felt easier and more relaxed with the course, the group and the teacher because being in a class room reminded me of all the years I had spent in education discussing things and reminded of all that.

I had heard of the power of positive thinking but the list of affirmations was mind blowing. We had to choose just one but it was difficult to pick a favourite as they were all so good. Others could be tried later on. As I have mentioned above though this turned out to be the most difficult thing on the course to do.

For some reason I likened the process of learning to a kind of brain washing but better to describe it as imprinting on the subconscious! Without all the post it notes everywhere displaying the maxim I would simply have forgotten to remind myself even without the great need to remember because of the severity of the problem

We did a timetable of weekly activities and was surprised to note I was a lot more active than I had imagined: for some reason I got the impression I was feeling anxious for a lot less time and was reassuring that most of the time I was ok. I think I had thought the problem was a lot less frequent than my mind made it out to be.

Maslow's hierarchy of needs was very enlightening as was the impact of drinking too much on the brains functioning. I was asked by the tutor if I had heard of Maslow to which I replied no. Later when I was talking about the class to a support worker some of what Maslow had to say has been contested but this wasn't mentioned in the class and I was left confused and wondering why not.

Basically Maslows says that people need to progress up a ladder of self development one rung at a time. Safety needs and self esteem needs were two of the rungs but it occurred to me that frightening delusions and critical voices would affect these safety needs and esteems needs respectively. This had not occurred to the tutor and no solution to these obstacles was offered.

One year on I still have the cards of my wall reminding me that I can do anything if I practice enough one can master anything but I still don't think this has rubbed off on me yet. Other things included a weekly timetable of activities which still reminds me I am quite active a lot of the time.

I also think the memory of the new people I met on the course and interacted with has helped me a little: it is not just something I was able to do years ago but something quite recent. Once I had this confidence with people I began to consider the idea of voluntary work.

Voluntary work

It was suggested to me that I might want to do some
voluntary work to provide some structure to my day
and give a reason to be out and about. A meeting was
arranged with the voluntary work coordinator from
local hospital who outlined the possible benefits. These
included that there might be some social contact and
new people to meet and a change of environment to be
in.

He very cleverly picked out a place I might feel relaxed
and at home in – the local botanic Gardens. After a
couple of weeks of deliberating about this I agreed to
give it a try, for just an hour at first. Before that
however I got him to ring up and find out about the job
first to find out exactly what it is I was going to be
doing. My main worry was that I might not have the
stamina to do something repetitive and that I might not
be meticulous enough for the job.

The next thought was would this affect my benefits and
place in Sheltered Accommodation but I was assured it
would not. That was a great relief! With this knowledge
in mind I was more willing to give it a try though with
the governments new deal for disabled people in mind I
still had a few doubts at the back of my mind.

My next thought was what if I had a panic attack while
I was up there and how would I cope with that? Having
had a few cach day after I had the advice about
voluntary work this thought was uppermost in my
mind. Then some happened to change this perception –
I had a social outing with a friend during which I did

not feel nervous and I began to have a more open mind about it.

Then doubts entered my mind again: I was a bit sceptical about any supposed benefits and thought to myself that I find it a bit monotonous typing stuff into a database all afternoon and even that it would do my head in! This time it took a push from my parents - something more forceful than the support from mental health services!

Then it struck me what the problem was: after another bout of fear I was reminded that it would be impossible to be somewhere other than home in order to cope with it much less being able to concentrate. Then once the fear had worn off I quickly forgot the experience and began to take the idea of voluntary work once more. I went through several cycles of this and ended up not knowing what to do!

The answer to this was to do a taster session lasting about an hour to see what it would be like, though I still tempted to scrap the whole project. Maybe the monotony could be overcome by practice? In the end this opportunity fell through as it was an old advertisement.

I started to consider the next alternative: working in the shop at a local museum. Would I be able to serve customers? I had some experience of bar work and wondered if that would help. On seeing the shop there was too much produce to assimilate...

There was no compulsion to do this and in the end I opted not to. The problem was that I was not able to formulate a goal which I think might have helped sway me in the direction of doing this. When life is aimless there does seem much point and to reiterate as my support worker said that can only come from you...

Yet there is still a valuable lesson here about the possible therapeutic value of voluntary work and that was only one way to find out about this and that was to give it a try.

Inside the Schizophrenic Mind

At this point I feel it necessary to introduce the schizophrenic context of my anxiety problems. Why am I so anxious? The problem is that thinking that I am responsible for 9/11 this thought is often at the back of my mind. The struggle I have is to keep active so that I do not think about it in the presence of other people. The reason being that if other people discern this in my thinking I might be punished for it.

While out and about I have to make conscious efforts not to think about this and to think about something else instead. It has been helped by going to places of interest, by having conversation, enjoyable food and shopping and many other things. All of this stops my mind drifting onto the subject of 9/11 and what might happen.

All the time I have had to contend with this problem I have been subconsciously afraid of my thinking reverting back to this delusion. I was hoping to socialise myself into not doing this – that with sufficient practice I would get used to thinking about other things and to overcome my associations that certain places reminded me of it. Places that I had a fear rush or panic attack when these thoughts came to my mind. I would remember the delusion through the fear associated with the place and then the terror comes back.

I was never convinced that this was possible or even worth trying: after all why take a risk like that? The mental health professionals and my family took a different view – that staying in my room would have such a negative impact on my life that it had to be helped. This did not persuade me initially.

The trials and tribulations I have had trying to go out and not think of 9/11 form a significant part of this book. I have taken risks in the context of my delusions by doing this though although it has required some courage to coexist with the fear rather than simply run away from what I was experiencing.

A nurse at the day unit told me that the two best ways of dealing with schizophrenia are to confront the fear at some times and distract yourself at others. The therapy of getting out and about involves a bit of both I was distracted by the various activities this involved and had to lesser extent overcome some of my fears about going out as well.

Mainly what follows is an account of how I have tried to distract myself by shopping, eating out, conversation, going out holiday and a number of other things (although it does look more like graded exposure to things that were frightening me). The fear never went away but my ability to distract myself gradually improved and I became a bit more functional in a way I first thought best to avoid at all costs.

The overall aim was to be able to go out without my subconscious mind worrying about what might happen if I did. This was a very difficult change to try to effect but I eventually tried to see if I could and sort to balance the benefits with the risks. I think what also comes through is how incredibly restrictive life with schizophrenia is, when even going to the local store becomes an obstacle.

This problem has dominated the symptoms of my schizophrenia and has dominated my life with the illness during the past five years. For this reason it is necessary to try to get across what life is like living like this I have described these problems in much detail below. This is not an account of overcoming fear but of trying to take your mind off schizophrenia and of socialising into these environments so that eventually the fear would wear off.

After a while I began to question more why I was so frightened when out and about and to do this I had to look at what I was thinking. I previously avoided doing this because I thought it was dangerous in the context of the delusions I was having.

My brain was telling me to continue getting out and about as a way of distracting my thought about being responsible for 9/11. If the thought of responsibility was confirmed then a punishment seemed likely. All the same I began to analyse and eventually felt quite comfortable doing this even though the thought of 9/11 was so frightening.

I began to notice that the fear it caused set my brains survival computer racing, constantly analysing about 9/11 and thinking I was being watched by people who could read my mind. Once I started to calm down this kept my mind quiet.

The problem seemed to me to be how to keep my mind quiet at these times and it seemed a number of strategies from the exposure approach to a then new psychological 'compassion focused' therapy might be relevant. This compassion approach is described below.

One was to practice the breathing, do the safe place imagery and compassionate self image when I was out and about. I noticed that the fear was being triggered by a cognition or thought about 9/11 and that this in turn would trigger the delusion.

It seemed sensible to calm down first and to prevent the delusion in the first place. If I kept calm then the technique might be applied to being in places where the associations of fear and danger were strongest.

After a while I didn't think these techniques were having much effect and I noticed how my brain began to handle the problem on its own.

I found I was keeping a grip on myself and tensing up until I could find a solution hoping in the way I would answer an essay question and that I could use these skills and instincts to find a solution. I was absorbing the information and storing it in my memory until a solution could be found.

This too was a way of grasping at straws because my brain flipped out and didn't know what else to do. My mind would react to other people with nasty thoughts about them and I felt people who saw this were threatening me back, or so I thought. This kept my brains threat system building.

During these outings the time seemed to fly and brain started thinking it would help the years to go by and not to drag so that being dead one day the CIA couldn't find me. This thought did occur to me from time to time but only on occasion did I take it seriously.

Another response was to naturalise being in a safe place where I had a homely feel about it. Often I would go somewhere that had good memories from before the illness and felt that I belonged in such places. This helped me blend into the crowd and stopped me feeling that I was being noticed whilst there. It helped switch my brain off and to calm down.

Often my adrenalin would be flowing and I would have a suppressed panic attack during which I kept trying to look normal. Staying in situ and waiting to calm down often got me through these moments during which I felt quite visible. I kept trying to distract my mind with something to stop it producing noticeable thoughts.

Something similar seemed to be happening during the time I spent indoors. I felt my mind was still being read and it set off lots of thinking to avoid them discerning any thoughts about 9/11. This was helped by keeping busy indoors, socialising by spending time with friends and family, travel and focusing on other things like music and film in an attempt to calm down and avoid my mind thinking about anything that might be dangerous.

I think I was focused on the experience of fear to the same effect, hoping in very difficult circumstances to get through life with the illness as quickly as possible, knowing too that if I could get over the feeling of fear this would make life much easier instead.

I also began to question what my motivations were for getting out and about (rather than simply doing what I was told by the CPN). Sometimes I had quite a positive sense of motivation that once I got out and calmed down the outings were really quite pleasant, something that made me again feel that I would enjoy voluntary work.

At other times I thought or at least hoped that getting out might lead to the goal of being able to do this without fear and that the graded exposure of different places might build towards this. Mostly though even while I had this hope I didn't feel I would get that far and it was enough merely to get out and about even while still feeling the fear.

Once I calmed down in the various places I went to the experience wasn't too bad and after I practised this a lot I felt this would be OK even if it never improved beyond this. That kept me motivated to keep trying the outings and even after the support worker help was finished. I kept practicing this with friends and family and began to think it was easier in their company despite the professional help.

A chain reaction

Then I got to thinking again. Why did I think people were reacting to them when I was out and about? It seemed to be that when I was getting paranoid and under the spot light I suddenly became more aware of my surroundings and started to notice the other people and being nervousness this made me visible.

So I tried to study the process by visualising what happened during my outing while being safe at home. I began to realise one thought or event led to another and started to create a chain reaction. I wonder whether it might be possible that once I isolated each stage in this chain it have been possible to arrest the process at each point.

Getting out of the car to go to my local shopping mall felt like abandoning somewhere safe and seeing the entrance to the Mall brought back memories of the last visit and the nerves that caused me.

Once inside the shop I felt highly visible and that my nerves made me conspicuous. This felt a lot like stage fright and I had to hurry through the shop and into the Mall. Once there I began to relax as the people were passing me by and not watching me.

I just assumed they were looking at other things like shop windows and looking around briefly would confirm this. However this safety assumption would not last as thoughts and memories of 9/11 would at some point start to drift into my mind. At this point I would get frightened and think that someone would discern this. That made me begin looking round for help and notice other people.

Then it struck me: people don't like to be noticed when out and about. It was no wonder they reacted to me doing this. I thought I was just being delusional and paranoid but in fact some of this could be actually happening. My psychologist concurred with me on this point and felt like I had distinguished between the real and the imaginary.

Then the row of dominoes started to topple one by one: I was suddenly aware of some sort of thought of danger. Thoughts are cognitions and I began to recognise by looking at other people that I was in peril. At the same time my memories would become activated by the sense of danger and the thoughts about 9/11 would come to the front of my mind.

Thinking people could perceive my thoughts they would start to recognise that I was thinking about 9/11. They may spot this and so I had the thought of 9/11 being broad cast to other people and this would be networked back to the CIA eventually by people telling other people. What was I to do?

Being schizophrenic and having occasional insight I then had another coping strategy. Once I got to the point of flipping out my reptile brain (where the brain focuses on self defence and counter attacking thoughts) came into play as I people were reading my mind. I began to deliberate hold in my mind the thought that I was schizophrenic. At this point people I hoped the people observing would think I was mad and so not connect me with the terrorist attacks I believed I was responsible for.

My mind began to be defensive and I tried to run away from the immediate situation and go inward while simultaneously to try to devise a solution to the problem that people were discerning I was responsible for 9/11. None of this worked but eventually when the thoughts subsided I gradually became aware of my surroundings again and things returned to normal.

So how was I supposed to stop this chain reaction? I began to analyse what might be done at each stage of the process and was able to draw up a series of coping strategies that could be used in sequence depending on what happened at each stage of the chain reaction. If one strategy didn't work then I had a back up plan and another back up plan and so on. This stopped me being so frightened at each point in the chain when something didn't work well I was reassured there was something else I could do that would help the anxiety. It helped me put up with the anxiety for longer when put and about.

My psychologist told me that nerves were triggers by an organ in the brain called the amygdala and this opens up the back of the brain where our fight/flight and survival responses are located. I recognised that I was having some cognition of danger my amygdala was clicking backwards and this was setting my reptile going. Could the process be arrested by my three step coping strategy?

My first thought here was if I could stop my amygdala clicking backwards, say by using aromatherapy oils, breathing to relax or safe place imagery (all things I covered with the psychologist) that would prevent the reptile brain triggering off its chatter and might stop me flipping out. At the confidence class we were told to take lavender when out and about and this was also a very effective way of keeping calm.

If I could not keep calm using all of these techniques and still became frightened then a second strategy became important which was to put into practice what the support worker had been trying to help with. Namely that instead of stopping the fear one might have to coexist with it instead. This was a way of preventing me from running from the place that had brought the fear on.

Finally if I got to the last stage in the chain and began to flip out then it was easy enough to go back to the car (which for me represents what psychologists call defended space) until I calmed down and was able to return to the frightening place.

After numerous attempts of doing this the strategy of keeping calm didn't seem to be working so I began to analyse more. I large part of the anxiety seemed to connected with memory. After years of building up associations of fear with certain places my brain my psychologist explained had been wiring neurons together and forming brain pathways which meant some rewiring was necessary.

Like any traumatic experience like that of a difficult childhood the memory of it could simply be erased by the therapeutic process of talking it though with the therapist. That would help remove my memories which were at the base of my reactions to certain places and overcome some of the psychological barriers to going out. The problem here was that if I continued to experience fear when practicing the exposure approach this would form new memories and circuits and that these associations would become psychologically.

Exposure to Fear

After a while a further development in my therapy was suggested by my CPN. It began with a question again as to what exactly was going through my mind to make me anxious. I replied I thought people were reading my thoughts. This is also something that Sandy Jeffs has experienced as she says in her excellent book *Flying with Paper Wings* so my case is not unique.

Thinking about 9/11 when out and about was to me something other people could detect when the thoughts about it ran through my mind. One they noticed this I began to worry if they would tell other people who would then pass the message on until it reached someone in authority. Once that happened I thought they would punish me in some indescribable terrible fashion.

With the support worker then another more immediate and personalised approach was to be tried. Sitting in a public place or walking through a supermarket or a store I began to feel people were aware of my presence. More than that if they were sitting in a cafe as opposed to passing them in a supermarket I began to feel I was being talked about.

The support worker being someone I trusted was able to question whether what they were saying was actually about me or just being some general conversation they were having. The more we practised this the more authoritative her reassurances became and the more I was able to question what I was thinking.

I got used to her reassurances and started to rely on them. I began to feel a little more confident again. Once she realised this it became important to try and get out about by myself so as not to create a relationship of dependency and it was re-emphasized that we must do work on getting out and about by myself.

I could hear the certainty in the support workers voice and she made eye contact while she was reassuring me. This made what she was saying more convincing and I began to trust her more and more. That trust was again built up once I heard what she had to say about the situation of being talked about.

The support worker continually posed the question was what I was hearing was actually connected with me being next to them or about someone else entirely? I was hearing one thing and thinking something else. The logic in this situation became very powerful and I was able to challenge my thinking. The was a stark contrast between the two possibilities and the support worker was on hand to reinforced the emphasise the differences.

So this worked because I was able to compare my thoughts with their chatter. Although I was thinking they were talking about me I could develop insight based on this evidence because once I actually listened to what they were saying I could tell it was not connected with me being there and most have been about someone or something else. Insight is a key goal for dealing with schizophrenia and delusions and I will return to this below when I describe my experiences of cognitive behavioural therapy.

For example if I was thinking about fish and the conversation I was overhearing was about cars then I felt I was not being reacted to. I could compare the thoughts in my head (which were also telling me that I was being talked about by other people) with what I was actually hearing. The hope was the more I was able to challenge my delusions in this way it would get easier and easier to go out without being frightened.

This approach proved to be a tricky business because for example they were talking about Coronation Street or something in the news I would immediately associate with that because another one of my delusions was that I was being talked about on television or causing events in the world which were being reported. Such conversation might have been deliberate because I was there and was being talked about deliberately to frighten me?

Most conversation I picked up was just people talking about their own lives just like what was displayed on a soap opera and because I identified with characters in these shows I felt they were repeating my thoughts again. It was like having my mind broadcast over the air ways or with the immediate vicinity of the cafe or shop. These made me very uncomfortable and I constantly tried not to think of 9/11.

The support worker very sensibly said to me that they went even looking in my direction let alone noticing I was there. There was less emphasis on whether mind reading was actual and possible and more on trying to reassure me that I wasn't being noticed. Again she said that they were simply engaged in conversation and not talking about a subject that had anything to do with me or 9/11.

Often though the delusional thinking was not directly connected with people talking about me but instead it was more a vague feeling I got that other people were aware of my presence. This was more difficult to challenge because the thought could not be dispelled by listening to what they were saying. It occurred to me that just because I was able to challenge the idea I was being talked about verbally that I was also picking up of vibes from other people and so it might be that I was getting false despite reassurances from my support worker.

At this point it appeared that it wasn't so much about what they said but more that they were reacting to my in giving out bad vibes because I was there. As I listened there seemed to be something not entirely normal about what I was hearing. For example I thought people were raising their voices because I was sat next to them or their intonation was deliberately contrived.

Nevertheless my support worker thought it fruitful to press ahead with this approach. She drafted a sheet which recorded place and time and I had to record what and when I thought this to be happen. It was something I had to do every day although this meant getting out and about by myself. Then I had to try to question what I thought was happening by writing whether the evidence support my interpretation.

It was first necessary to get the idea of what I was being asked to do. The support worker asked if something came up to me and stated all of this thinking described here would I believe them? How would someone else view what I was saying? I said I would view such a person to be delusional. That was a good start I was told.

After that I began to again record such instances. As the weeks went by I began to compile a lengthy list with hundreds of examples. The hope was that after doing the same thing many times I would begin to question what I was thinking, to undermine the beliefs I had. This is an on-going process in my therapy and the outcome is still undecided.

My CPN too asked how long I had thought that people had been reading my mind about 9/11 and I said about five years. Trying to develop some insight into my delusion again he said why has nothing happened to me so far? Surely if I had caused 9/11 some action would have been taken straight away. A good question I thought: I said that eventually something would be done about but could explain why they would wait – it was just what I believed to be the case.

Subsequently the support worker decided to accompany me to meeting of the cognitive behavioural therapy whose job it was to develop insight. The outings were narrated to the CBT specialist and he thought he could usefully build upon and focus on these experiences of challenging my delusions. Unfortunately as we have seen in my essay on CBT above when we began to discuss my experiences of this the insight was difficult to develop and I the end I felt that there was only so much insight that a person could have.

Coexisting with the fear

I have often wondered whether this title bears some relation to what Susan Jeffers calls face the fear and do it anyway. But that phrase begs a key point about what we were trying to do by going out. It was frightening but the fear did not necessarily put me off as I could still do it even when frightened. It wasn't necessary to stop the fear but coexist with it. This was the second strategy in the chain reaction.

To coexist with the fear I had to stay mindful of my surroundings and not to run from them. Often being mindful only occurred when I began to calm down and became more aware of my immediate surroundings. Often too my mind was somewhere else when thinking about delusions or listening to voices all day. It was quite difficult to simply be in the here and now and even going for a walk did not distract me enough to enjoy the nature and the sunshine. I was simply too preoccupied most of the time.

Once I began to watch myself and be mindful of what was happening to me I began to notice differences in my reactions depending on situation. My brain would flip out in differing ways depending on the trigger but I could still force myself to be in that situation and not go back to the car or my flat, depending on where I was. This took some practice depending on where I was.

Watching the television was one instance. Here the fear was closely bound up by the political context that millions of people were watching a catastrophe I was responsible for. This was one major fear I had and coexisting with fear of this magnitude seemed to be the most difficult.

Another problem occurred when passing people on the rail way line. Suddenly I was not anonymous but in a social situation. I didn't know how to react to this either and I was certainly not trying to be mindful of the problem. At the shopping mall these social situations hardly ever arose but here the fear was generated in a different way. But it is the coexisting with the TV example that I want to concentrate on as this caused the most direct and challenging exposure to my terrors.

It was recommended by the cognitive therapist that I watched a video about 9/11 with my support worker on hand to provide reassurance. I had to coexist with the fear of doing this. But at this point the experience went over my head and this kept happening when out and about as well. Mostly though I could notice things in my environment but the rest of my brain was reacting differently.

I was so frightened of the TV that I was not altogether able to focus on what I was watching and my mind would run from it so mindfulness was again recommended as the solution to it. To be mindful and afraid at the same time. The support worker told me to be aware it was there and even that I was there too.

At first glance my brain was recognising and remembering danger. The thought of danger flashed up in the front of my mind. My eyes widened at watch I was watching. I could barely believe what I was seeing was real and still the magnitude of it made me flip out.

In fact of being responsible for 9/11 was so unbelievable I could stare at it with a strange fascination and not react to it with fear. Later my eyes became glazed and my vision became hazy. I was so identified with what I was seeing I lost my sense of physical space between me and the television.

My subconscious was stirring warning me of the danger and I had a nervous reaction. Once I achieved some focus I still had the impression my senses were being by passed by what I was watching and this seemed to stop noticing what I was looking at.

I was attempting to identify with the video instead of engaging with it. I was so identified I forgot I was there. Transfixed by what I was watching my reptile brain remained silent and stopped trying to analyse what I was watching, trying to problem solve a way of calming down.

I had a look of horror in my eyes and a mocked sense of shock and the same time my brain was recognising the enormity of what I believed I had caused with 9/11. Only occasionally did this produced a subconscious reaction and my brain desperately tried to think of something else.

Instinctively my brain tried to run in any direction it could in order to focus and think about anything else. It conjured mental images or lines of thought but was not able to latch on to any of this so as to be distracted from or otherwise to stop thinking about 9/11.

At the same time another part of mind was recognising that it could not let the thought of 9/11 go as it had to do something to solve the problem that I might be punished for it.

I had to accept responsibility for what I believed had happened but also had to find a way to avoid punishment that might be acceptable to the voices which were constantly watching the mental turmoil.

My intellectual faculties were still functioning and I was trying to use them to analyse the delusion much the same as I have done to some extent in writing this essay. Again this did not help with being mindful as I was thinking about something else.

The problem was partly to keep my senses and feel afraid simultaneously. Far from being mindful of the fear which was there in my immediate surroundings my mind tried to run away from it mentally even when I was forced to stay put physically. In the end coexisting with the fear seemed very difficult to do.

A New Psychiatrist

After more than ten years with one consultant I was transferred to see a new psychiatrist. The new doctor was very experienced and at least as expert as the one I had before. There was some difference in style and I was in and out to see the new consultant very quickly compared to the in depth approach of the last psychiatrist.

I thought this would mean starting again from the beginning and narrating my whole history including when I had been in hospital and what medication I had been on during different phases of my illness. I also thought it best to keep my CPN on hand to answer all these questions but instead he was most interested in the current phase I was going through and did not ask for a psychiatric history.

Nevertheless he expressed some interest in my past writing and the radio interview I did with my family. "We like to hear first-hand accounts" he said. In particular he wanted to know about what the symptoms were and how severe they appeared and here my past experiences were interesting to him even though in most patients the same symptoms are present during the whole life time of being ill

I told him I had been through different phases during my twenty years of illness including running around the country side trying to evade auditory hallucinations, having pain hallucinations and been too frightened to go out in case people were spying on me.

The detail of the experience of these phases meant that they were very different as varied from wandering around the countryside in a daze not knowing where I was to what it is like being trapped in a room for a year and not going out. Occasionally doctors will take a case history and this is included in part of their training and I think my history such as it is would have been very interesting to them.

I then tried to explain that I heard voices all day long and had terrifying delusions. The voices blamed me for causing 9/11 but I said I would have believed this anyway had the voices been silenced. He very quickly understood that the illness was mainly an anxiety/fear problem more than anything else and with that I could only agree.

I had to give the new doctor a few examples of how my illness manifested itself and this provided a good opportunity to present some quite graphic examples. One thought was that every time I went upstairs in my family home a picture of my niece always seemed to have a new expression on its face every time I went passed it and that this expression changed each time depending on whatever mood I was in.

Another concerned the fact that schizophrenics often think they are being talked about on televisions. During my exposure approach to the illness I was led by a support worker into an electrical retailers where I was surrounded by televisions. The result was to multiply the effect of each broadcast on each television set with lots and lots of voices (from the televisions) talking about me everywhere I looked. It was like having a hundred people talking about me at once and I had to run out of the shop.

Earlier in my illness I had a another good example. This was another variation on the theme that schizophrenics are being talked on television. Believing I was responsible for wars and diseases I felt like a social outcast and people were watching television in every house I passed as a method of keeping me away from them. This was a kind of punishment for the bad things I believed I had   caused in the world.

As for severity a could only make a number of remarks about that. I said as above that I could be frozen in fear to the point of not being able to move, my metabolism racing at a hundred miles per hour and being full of adrenalin to the point of being in physical pain. That was about as graphic as I could get whilst probably not able to be able to go into very great detail about it but it was enough for the new doctor anyhow.

I also said I had visual hallucinations such as when I went home the picture of my niece on the hall way wall always had a different expression on its face every time I walked past it. My CPN remarked it was very unusual to experience visual as well as auditory explanations at the same time.

I think it is true that a new broom sweeps keen and after hearing about my symptoms he had some new suggestions regarding my medication. Different doctors all have their favourite medications, including things they won't touch, and mine was no exception. The new doctor wouldn't prescribe a benzodiazepine and also wanted to try a combination of my current medication with something newer (actually abilify).

Once I had described my anxiety causing symptoms he asked me closely about my mood. I replied I was generally too frightened to have low mood. I don't know if that was a correct answer but I wasn't put on an anti-depressant specifically for this though I would still be put on one anyway to help cope with the anxiety.

The new doctor explained there were a lot of different anti-depressants he could try and that I would be seen at regular intervals to monitor their impact. That too came as a surprise to me as it had been a few years since I saw my last consultant and had regularly saw my CPN instead.

So over the preceding months I was introduced to a lot of tablets I had never heard of including pregabaline, mirtazapine (his favourite) and sertraline none of which really had any impact on my nerves. These drugs brought back images of the mental health system many people will be familiar with because it means putting up with new side effects and trying to guess if there was any improvement.

I was quickly rushed off the first one when it brought me out in rash. Why this was so I don't know. I was then told to record in a diary about whether there was any improvement. I found my condition did fluctuate a bit though I also had a few mental battles trying to think whether there had been any improvement or not overall.

This never really raised my hopes. I guess I had seen so many people with so many drugs changes I got to thinking If there was going to be any improvement I would believe it when I see it. In my case after trying his five different drugs he said he had done all he can but I was left wondering whether a new psychiatrist would have preferred something different.

I know a lot of people will say such and such a drug worked for me and to try to encourage some optimism about this and I do try to keep an open mind but I think this can be hard some times when I have seen so many different doctors and approaches all of which only work in a about a third of cases (eg anti-psychotics and CBT) that I have more hope for the talking treatments on the whole.

Tertiary Psychoses

After a further period of time the anxiety began to increase again despite all this apparent progress. It was decided by my CPN to refer me to a more psychological approach and I was nominated to the Tertiary psychoses team at my local (mental) hospital.

My first reaction to this was what does tertiary psychosis mean which I am sure will be the readers first reaction as well. Apparently drugs are primary, cognitive behavioural therapy is secondary and psychology tertiary. I got to the point of thinking well if this is the last thing to try it will be just my luck if it doesn't work!

Curiously enough I had never heard of this approach before despite having been in the mental health system for twenty years and I think a lot more should have been done to publicise it. Especially since the illness is treatment resistant to the latest drugs (they still only cure a third of cases with olanzapine and respridone) and CBT likewise only cures 29%.

I was told by the tertiary psychoses team that I would be referred to group work entitled Compassion focused therapy. Again I wondered what that meant. It was explained that by developing compassion we can soothe the fear caused by schizophrenia and feel better about ourselves when we have voices that criticise us. This was a lengthy process as I shall now have to summarise.

At the first meeting we introduced ourselves to the other members of the group. The friendliness of the group was essential to relaxing with each other and showing compassion to the other people. This was facilitated by provided tea and coffee and we tried to enhance the social environment by going to a coffee shop in our local town centre after the group to get to know each other better.

The subsequent sessions took the form of a taught course as at a college. There were handouts, a board and questions and members of which I was familiar with from Uni. This helped me relax further. And indeed some of the class consisted of research students to boot!

Teaching in the class covered a variety of different subjects and as 'the course' progressed I gradually came to understand it as a series of exercises that could be performed concurrently. My psychiatrist insisted that at some point it would all click into place but my progress in understanding the class and doing the exercises has progressed very slowly and I am currently eighteen months into this therapy. After the end of the group, which lasted for over six months, I had a short break and now see my psychologist on a one-to-one basis.

These exercises including breathing exercises (again), keeping a pleasure/gratitude diary, imagining myself in a safe place, having a compassionate self image, imaging a strawberry (I shall explain this later!), recording achievements, showing each other compassion in the group and a number of other things. In my case all this did not seem to be enough and so there was also some emphasis on trying with anti-depressants again alongside the psychology therapy.

The therapy in my case seemed to centre around the biological operation of the brains alarms system which we discovered was called the amygdala. Basically whenever the brain perceives a threat the amygdala responds and shuts down the frontal lobes and opens up the back part of the brain which computes our flight fight responses.

The effect of fear in this process is close down the frontal parts that deal with logical thought emotion creativity and even personality. The problem seemed to be therefore how to open up these parts of the brain again.

One way of doing this was practicing the pleasure diary and safe place imagery both of which caused some pleasure and I could feel this reacting in my frontal lobes. We learned on the course that neurons that fire together also wire together and I could feel that I was forming pleasure circuits in this area of the brain to the effect that my frontal lobes began to open up a little. Regular practice at this meant these circuits would build and build.

Ironically the more frightened responses the brain has to deal with means that circuits and neurons were also firing and wiring in the back part of the brain. Any threat that the brain has to deal with in life causes this response and a lot of emphasis in the class had to deal with childhood and other traumas.

These memories of anxiety which in my case were caused by an absent father in childhood could be overcome simply by knowing that these traumas purely exist as memories and don't affect any other influence on us. That fact was not obvious to me until it was pointed out and forms an important part of the therapy.

Another thought which occurred to me was that what would happen to me if I stopped using my occipital brain to deal with the threats caused by paranoid delusions and critical voices. The answer again was to open up the frontal lobes which is where we experience compassion and then to use this and the strength compassion gives the person to overcome the fear of the delusion and soothe the effects it has on us.

Compassion we learned connects us to other people emotionally and as such is the basis of friendship and relationships which in turn further strengthens us against the effects of threats caused by mental illness. The back part of the brain which we learned was reptilian closes the cooperative frontal lobes down in order to affect an instinctive fight flight response and so diminishes the emotional support we can get.

Compassion we learned is sensitivity to suffering and the consequent motivation to do something about it. It gives us the strength to cope with anxiety. However after two years of this therapy I have not completed the course and so cannot yet give an end to my experiences of anxiety.

One way of getting our frontal lobes to open up is to activate the pleasure circuits was to give aromatherapy oils a go. I can almost hear every ones reaction to this that essential oils are not powerful enough to calm schizophrenia but that is not the point.

I could feel the oils having the same effects on the pleasure circuits that I had also noticed from the safe place imagery. The point then was not primarily to relax but instead to experience pleasure in the frontal lobes.

Indeed the same effect could also be derived from after shaves and anything with a perfume and this became something I could combine with the safe place imagery too. Focusing on an object with all our senses (the object in this case was a strawberry) also helped the same end of opening up the front part of my brain.

I also learned that the amygdala was the brain emotional memory centre and that an experience of childhood trauma would clog it up so much that it was very difficult to click it forward. I pointed this fact out to the therapist since in my case there had been some emotional issues since childhood that were having, in biological terms, an impact on the therapy and we agreed to explore these at a later date.

This lead to an understanding of something else I had previously written about in part two of my book *The Stages of Schizophrenia*. Life before the illness seemed so much brighter and images from my past where much sharper. Everything else just seemed to be a blur after that.

The psychologist explained this was because the amygdala was also the brains emotional memory centre and the experience of being schizophrenic tended to dampen down our emotional awareness of life. The reason again was that it was not clicking forward as much as it should be.

This is the bare bones of the new therapy and according to the therapist it is more powerful than the breathing exercises and safe place imagery I was using to try and get out and about. It has given me much hope that my schizophrenia might one day be cured. Any one wishing to find out more about it should consult Paul Gilberts excellent book titled *The Compassionate Mind*.

Critical Voices

Hearing voices not just about 9/11 has also been a prominent experience of my illness and has been another major source of anxiety with schizophrenia. These voices have created problems other than getting out and about and as many people with schizophrenia will tell you what you hear when hallucinating can be very critical and once again to return to the main themes in this book that is frightening.

One particular distraction from hearing voices which is peculiar to my psychology is the fact I was, according to the voices, a loser. The voices began to criticise me for this and I began to slowly watch my main way of being distracted from the hallucinations was now being undermined and disappearing.

What is a loser I here you cry? In a nutshell it was an attitude to life that without success life on any other terms is not worth it. It makes the rich feel guilty and the poor feel their lives are worthless. Naturally being a loser carries a strong stigma and so as Fleetwood Mac sing about the lives of people in this category that they must: "pick your path and now pray."

One example (and there are many) would be Ozzy Ozbournes song "Secret Loser" which contains the lines "I can understand that what you see you think is real, couldn't every take my soul cos it isnt there to steal". Another is by Sheryl Crowe "If it make you happy it can't be that bad, then why the hell are you so sad". Further notable examples are to be found the Albums of the Corrs and I am sure the reader will be thinking of others now too.

The effect of the voices was to try and get me to realise that this psychology was a bar to a more normal self development. They were slowly purging my mind of this way of' loser thinking' in exactly the same way as in the critical pop culture has done in the quotes above.

So I keep playing songs that are more sympathetic or have good memories in order to fight the process that being a loser is something bad as the voices seemed to indicate. Eventually though the voices seemed like they were going to win out on this and I could not in the end resist the influence of the hallucinations in this way.

For me though this battle has been the major focus of my distractions from my schizophrenia and I am now getting the subconscious thought that what will happen when it ends? What will happen without this major distraction from feeling responsible for 9/11 disappears? Will my other delusional thoughts be magnified?

Having grown up with this psychology there is a lot of emphasis on what had been achieved materially and intellectually in my life and being a loser tends to over identify and over value such things. The emphasis on materialism had provided another distraction as when I went to the shopping Mall and the intellectual overemphasis has resulted in my writing and research. What was going to happen to me if it all stopped?.

Being criticised about all this from the voices and society and even our own internal self critic makes me re-examine every instance of this loser thinking especially, for instance, was I right to have over identified with the material side of life and whether I should accept the opposing values? I began to have a long argument with the voices.

That made me retreat into memories of the past when I was free from such pressures but it also in turn set me thinking that I was seeing everything in my past through the eyes of being a looser. I had many emotional memories of feeling like this loser person for example that I was rationally dissatisfied with my lot. I felt that I had been seeing everything them under the aspect of how they appeared to me as a loser instead of how they might have normally have appeared from the viewpoint of the observing voices.

These voices were particularly good at undermining all of this through exploiting my nice side and they said I was selfish and should be grateful for what I had rather than wanting things I didn't have. Again I found myself engaged in a long battle with myself about whether they were right or not partly because I believed my loser standpoint to be right.

Eventually though the criticism began to take root in my mind and I began to engage in a constant battle with myself. The struggle became internal instead of with the voice. Invoking the memories became to seem less and less justified and I had to let go of them and this began to erase the associations, memory by individual memory, attachment by attachment and also thought by thought.

I made the memories and materialistic situations into part of me and wouldn't let them go in the face of all this. Eventually though under much pressure from the voices I was forced to severe these attachments and I felt like I was being stripped bare. Once Gone I would be defenceless (and without distraction).

So I tried to submerge myself into my associations with movies, music and household tasks to escape from the problem. This was difficult because as I have referenced popular culture is so full of such criticism. In any case I rapidly became bored with most of it as when not able to watch TV the few parts of the culture I could listen to were repeated ad nauseum. This plan didn't work out.

One by one the memories and attachments were being erased. My mind had been shaped according to this psychology and as I have indicated my thought patterns and identity had also been influenced. Losing these associations felt not only like stripping my identity but also losing the way I had previously and fundamentally thought about my life.

I had lived this way for so long it not only felt natural and normal but I had lost awareness that I had even been thinking along these lines at all. I certainly was not aware that I was a loser and once the voices started telling me about all thus it all it came as a bit of a shock. I was also suddenly aware of all the pop psychology that stigmatised it too.

What I had thought to be normal life came to feel not as a natural experience but a way of thinking and engaging with it in ways that had been imprinted on me as a child and that were actually not socially acceptable. As my psychologist reminded me this was not my fault but the voices didn't care about this.

All my life memories, emotional ones in particular, came to seem to be just an imprint. An attitude to life rather than lived experience. I began to change my mind about life. The problem was having grown up like this the associations they were so strong and varied that they have been difficult to sever. They had seemed to seem to be a very strong defence against thinking about other things like my delusions in this way.

It was then that the voices starting criticising what they saw as the envy involved with being a loser, born out of what they saw as my relative inability to perform better academically, they continued to criticise it and try to erase my writing skills too.

So they then began to criticise my academic skills and undermine my confidence even with what I had written about mental health. Interpretive questions about my writing began to preoccupy me and the more I doubted the more the voices began to question that I was envious of more intelligent people. That mirrored my underlying psychology of being a looser and put even more pressure on me to change my attitude to life in the ways outlined above.

I think here the voices have questioned my intelligence because they tell me if I was to do something socially useful they might let me off with being responsible for 9/11. So the fact they began to question my intelligence, education and writing was both frightening to me and made the voices even more critical.

So sooner or later I would be confronting the delusion without being able to escape from it. Then what would happen? My coping strategies might have gone. Then I would probably be more likely to be held responsible? Having total and continual exposure to my delusions is thankfully something I have been able to avoid in this way so far as it keeps the voices talking about something else but that as they say would be another story.

Being absorbed

In this essay I want to further detail and examine the important matter with my schizophrenia, just described in the last essay, that I have been able to avoiding psychotic thinking through the operation of other parts of my psychology.

Instead of my delusions dominating my mind I have been able providing an alternative focus in my life and from there to mostly avoiding confrontation with and overcoming my delusions. I could overcome the fear of schizophrenia while still having and ignoring the original psychotic thought.

My thoughts often involved association with the physical environment and intellectual and emotional thoughts about how I see my life progressing even when ill. These are clearly important things and the mind can focus on them quite easily.

Other thoughts for example involved reminders of a sense of place and the good memories I have of certain places as for example were I feel more relaxed or happy. For instance where I go to the local shopping Mall I can feel quite at home and more connected with parts of me that identify with the place.

My brain has also been trying to get involved with my surroundings and experiences even when at home because it knows I can stop thinking about 9/11 by doing to. This also helps pass the time until either a solution to the illness presents itself or else sadly sometimes to burn the time away until I get to the end of my life without suffering too much.

This can also be an act of desperation. So at the other times I will examine parts of my life that I can analyse needlessly, such as my taste in fashion, in order so to pass the time. Feeling I was being watched by the voices I had to think of something else in order not to be punished by them. My brain was doing this by itself without any pushing from me.

My brain can spend a lot of time doing this without schizophrenia and getting control over this activity can be quite difficult because it is being subconscious driven by the fear I have. We can for example spend a lot of time daydreaming but with schizophrenia all this proves a welcome distraction as it stops me being afraid a lot of the time.

Occasionally though the thoughts about 9/11 do still enter my mind in spite of the distraction. They can drift into my thoughts just as easily as other subjects. My strategy was certainly not effective as much as would like.

So far I have mentioned that I could get lost in my thinking about something so I don't notice my surroundings or alternatively so absorbed in my environment whether at the Mall or at home as in front of the TV that I forget I am there and this has helped me with distraction most of the day.

What I don't understand is how the nervy threatening feeling of being responsible for 9/11 which I am always conscious of at the back of my mind allows me to get lost in this way. Shouldn't I be automatically preoccupied with it more? It seemed to me that one part of my mind was thinking about one thing while another was aware of the danger.

The three main preoccupations I had were over identification with my environment, day dreaming about certain things and self immersion involving introspective thinking about myself. Only at certain points did I wake up and realise what I was doing. I could get lost in my thinking to the point I was only peripherally aware of my delusions. Again the voices were criticising me for doing this.

Another way of getting lost was to bury my head in academic work and writing including writing this book. This time I was more in control of what my mind was doing. I told myself that I needed to pursue the goals and keep with the motives with this work in order to fulfil what the voices demanded of me in terms of atonement.

So I launched hook line and sinker into education to pursue the goals as the voices wanted. I began to understand that the threat drove my subconscious mind to pursue education and started moulding my conscious brain to measure up to be able to do this.

I could see my mind visibly forming and shaping tangibly to the task in hand. The threat system in my reptile brain was gearing up to the challenge linking it to my perceptions, creativity, logic and intuitions and other relevant parts of the mind. I used what I was engaging with to keep my delusional worries at the subconscious level.

I came to rely on my thinking, affirming its correctness so as to generate some faith and confidence that I could achieve the goals set by the voices. When the voices started to criticise me for doing this they were able to generate some actual doubts about whether I could achieve what they wanted. After this the voices turned more nasty and I began to lose my intellectual interests as an immersive coping strategy.

I always had the fear my 9/11 delusion might intrude and didn't dare acknowledge to myself that the thought was there at the back of my mind. Analysing the thought itself might trigger a realisation that I was really the culprit and might be punished so it was only after a lot of thinking that I was able to analyse the thought itself and see if that provided a way of relaxing with it.

Then looking into my mind more I began to notice other mental processes coming into play. There were lots of drives in operation in my reptile brain prompted by the perception of threat. I began to see what was happening in my mind and after the voices criticised my drive motives for not succeeding. I then lost another aspect of my psychological and mental makeup which could have absorbed me into thinking about something other than 9/11.

All the time my mind was trying to pull in another direction to escape thinking about the truth in these beliefs but at the same time I was frightened that somehow my thoughts would betray me. This was equally true whether out and about or sat in my room. Just when one drive was erased another came along and I thankfully to some extent began to be absorbed in this inner analysis instead, even though its destructive mentally erasing consequences would have ended badly by erasing my motivations to study therein.

Then an idea occurred to me: would my thoughts really do this and was I worrying needlessly that this losing of my abilities might not actually happen? This was the first glimpse I had of a total picture of what was happening to me, since my mind had always tried to look elsewhere rather directly into itself and I had never up to this point ever dared or been able to do this seeing of myself.

There was the constant perception of threat in my reptile brain and this was so frightening it seemed more sensible to avoid the issue of whether to discern if there had been any threat at all in the ways I have described. I was merely assuming that my mind might drift onto the fact that I had caused 9/11 without questioning whether this might actually happen and whether it could be coped with if it did happen? It seemed easier to run away from thinking about it.

So I also had in my memory of the terror that I might be held responsible for 9/11 and in my thinking this worked to the same end of avoiding the issue and much of my brain began to instinctively rationally and emotionally to avoid the issue. The question again was could these successful avoidance strategies be dispensed with and this seemed a frightening possibility to try. That task is also for another book.

Adaption not distraction

Often then the usually recommended strategy of distraction is very difficult and the fear and perception of threat takes over. There are clearly limits to how effective this coping mechanism can be so again what happens when it fails?

The feeling of being highly visible makes my mind runaway from the people and yet at the same time produces a defensive strategy. At this point I only runaway mentally rather than physically and my mind tries to produces solutions. As I have said one is that I tell the people who become aware that I am responsible for 9/11 that this is a merely a schizophrenic delusion and hope this stops them observing me.

Yet this strategy is not full proof as I then start to think that they might get frightened of the fact that I am "a schizophrenic" and that makes me feel even more visible which in turn exacerbates and increases the original problem of anxiety. Usually this can get to the point of being so damaging that I have to remove myself physically and for example go back to the car as I have described.

Watching and knowing the detail of what happens has become a source of study and questioning for me and so I have asked what exactly are the triggers and how does my schizophrenic mind respond to them?

The more I study the more I realise that the triggers where very subtle. Often it was the perception of threat or flashback of fear when out and about. The more I kept generating negative responses to the various environments causing this the more I realised the triggers became more frequent and subtle. It took less and less powerful triggers to cause the same level of anxiety that I have described with my illness. This realisation nearly put me off going out again.

When out and frightened I stopped being distracted and was more consciously aware of my surroundings. I found myself trying desperately to control my own thoughts and to naturalise myself into the environment where ever I was. I had to impose some order on what was happening to me to get control over my reactions and return things to a feeling of and outward show of normality. On reflection this too seemed impossible.

Another consequence of these difficulties was that I began to lose associations of places and people that I remembered had felt safe before the illness. That affected my sense of self identity which admittedly had originally formed at times in my life when I was influenced by my loser psychology but I have said this was being in turn erased and undermined by the voices criticising me for being like this anyway.

By concentrating on my loser psychological associations to things and places where had a feeling of safety I was able to refocus my attention away from the observing people and voices away and from the issues of being responsible from 9/11. Most of the difficult times when out and about could be dealt with on this basis as the associations formed such a strong part of my self-identity.

This statement needs an example. As the Stone Roses sang about losers they absurdly think "there is a place for me anywhere". People with this psychology do think that statement. We become identified with environments that we do not belong to.

This carries a heavy stigma in popular culture as I have said with me this was added to by the critical voices so that this feeling of belonging somewhere together with the safe place coping strategy was beginning to be destroyed too.

Yet with schizophrenia it was reliance on this feeling of being identified in certain places that gets undermined by the experience of paranoia of being in them. If the original identification can be criticised as invalid it loses this feeling of safety and as the associations are destroyed, the psychological reaction of safety is further undermined.

This most visibly happened to me when I first became ill. I ran home when I first started to get symptoms and despite this my illness continued to deteriorate. Both the feeling of being at home and the experiences of the terrifying illness stayed with me and I can vividly remember both sets of feelings. Home and schizophrenia are for me both easily remembered and the illness spoilt my feeling of safety being there.

The more I tried to get out and about in safe places the more I was becoming ill in them too and again this spoilt the feeling of security again. This in turn has posed problems for the coping strategy of my psychologists i.e. that of imaging yourself in a safe place.

At this point we can throw the criticism of being a loser into the mix that that such a sense of place is not a valid attachment anyway and the effectiveness of the coping strategy is prevented when out. This outcome as with a lot of what has happened to me is peculiar to having this loser trait in the first place and may be relevant only in that context.

So this book has led me on a journey for from the problem of anxiety into my own schizophrenic mind and it is here that I will look for a solution next. So in my following books on this subject I will look into my thought patterns further and see if I can impose some further order on what I am thinking. That is going to be another subject.

Summing Up

Looking back a number of things stick in my mind and I think it possible to draw a number of conclusions. If I had to pick the most significant parts of this essay in summary what follows below is what spring most clearly to mind.

One is that at the outset what was uppermost in my mind was the fear and the different levels of fear in different places. When I began to observe and analyse more I began to understand what I was thinking and this came to help me in that I had in built coping strategies of distraction that made going out less of a problem.

That helped me realise the risk of going out was not as great as it first seemed and that with sufficient practice I could reduce and eventually eliminate the fear that this was causing. I hoped that the associations I could create in doing this would come to be more prominent for me and uppermost in my mind as compared to the fear it was generating.

There also was the need to keep pushing the boundaries for example the need to meet new people and then being pushed not to become dependent on this help. This has been a difficult issue for my support workers because the stress could have caused me to snap.

Another is that bottling out of doing one thing quickly leads to bottling out of doing something else. It weakens your resolve and often magnifies the problem of anxiety greatly and thinking like this can make me housebound. We end up making mountains out of molehills and that we cannot help ourselves.

However without challenging the fear things would never have improved so it was I think necessary to take the risk. Handled properly and by graded exposure some definite progress has been made although a complete remedy has not yet been effected using the approaches outlined here. Being able to do all this took a few years but it got there in the end.

Another area of improvement was that I stopped hitting the bottle so much after a period of being at home. Being at home was a lot more relaxing than the project I lived in even to the point that I occasionally thought it best to move back there. This helped me get off the drink and without this my drinking could have posed a serious health risk. Regrettably I could not get off the drink completely but still have still improved a lot.

Eventually the outings with my support worker got less frequent, which began by dropping our weekly Friday session and later by rescheduling our two hour Tuesday session to be fortnightly. Finally I decided it to call it a day saying I could practice getting out and about with friends and family and this is the stage I am currently still in.

Overall I have found it easier to be absorbed while at my family home and the homely project I live in (which by dcfinition is safer and more familiar) than getting out and about. Yet this has created the need to *push* myself to go out in the first place and again some places are safer and more familiar in the same way.

Living with this illness has greatly been helped by my ability to distract myself or as I call it being absorbed. When at home I can be completely immersed in the television or conversation with my friends and when out and about in all the familiar places and situations I have described above I can be almost completely immersed in my surroundings.

This has aided with passing the time so that I am not thinking about the illness the whole time and has helped take the pressure off a lot. I can have rejuvenating periods of relaxation despite the risk of cracking up and snapping at other times. I believe that if I was getting symptoms 24/7 my life would have been a lot harder.

I think the focus of this book too is that it also contains some examples of what the *experience* of schizophrenia is like and it has some graphic examples of what struggling with the illness and its various symptoms are like. Life with the illness *is* very difficult and in this book and I think I have given an account of that as an experience of what schizophrenic problems are like more than it is a book on anxiety management.

If there is a positive message in this book it is not that I have overcome this anxiety just through courage. Rather as I think I have learned to live with fear rather than stop the anxiety completely and that I think that life with schizophrenia is worth it despite the great struggles and great problems it creates.

Yet some courage has been involved. With milder levels of anxiety keeping busy and distracted has worked well but for more moderate levels there has to be some mind over matter. When the anxiety is at its worse there isn't really much I can do about it other remove myself from the situation causing it, getting back to sleep on the tablets or grasping at straws by trying to absorb myself into something else.

That question has led me to examine this underlying thinking and as I have described it has allowed me to concentrate on other things and has even come in useful in the most difficult sorts of situation. Yet often this aspect is peculiar to and my looser psychology so it maybe my case here is fairly unique in some ways. Nevertheless it has allowed me to cope with terror as much as anything else.

Another thing is that has given me hope much more recently is the compassion based theory. I can see what this therapy is trying to achieve and it makes a lot of sense as an approach to mental illness. Since it is something I can practice alongside the graded exposure and medication strategies I have found it valuable not to compartmentalise the essays written in this book. I have written much on this in *Schizophrenia Bulletin* and *Psychoses Journal* so anyone wishing to follow this story further should look there.

In the end it may be that getting out and about will eventually become easier as I know that when I practice doing this I do eventually calm down. That thought spurs me on to keep trying and to watch what happens. The hope is that after sufficient practice doing this the feelings of safety, relaxation and pleasure become longer and longer each time and that the feelings of fear will eventually and gradually go away.

That process keeps having set-backs because it can cause trauma. Instead of getting back and feeling refreshed associate the places I go to can result in experiencing trauma which puts me off going out ever again. But with careful thought and the passage of time these feelings can subside or be forgotten and I get back to a state of mind where i think these problems can be overcome.

The hope is to get back to a with a feeling of security, the same as before the illness. When out and about in the same places I used to go to before being ill the memory and association of the time before can be spoilt and I lose the feeling of familiarity and makes me feel safe. Yet these memories can be built upon by new experiences of being safe and the past and present experiences may become a powerful combination for getting out and about again and calming down as well at home and elsewhere.

A Message of Hope

What I have learned about life from my experience of anxiety has been very valuable. Suffering in this way has taught me much about the human condition and the trials that life can throw at you. Struggling in this was makes you a real person and allows some sensitivity and compassion for the sufferings of others throughout the world.

We can leave behind the shallow minds and materialism and grow as a person so that we become 'real people.' We can to some extent turn the experience from being something negative into something we can learn from.

We can realise life is often not a bowl of cherries and that we can stand up to some of our problems. Yet we can rely on help to do this rather than suffering the stigma that our weaknesses have driven us mad and we dont deserve or need help.

So when we can develop compassion for ourselves for example we generate empathy for others and our knowledge of people grows immensely. We feel connected to others going through difficult times and our knowledge of the human condition and its problems grows too.

If we can cope with schizophrenia we can cope with almost anything. I think life with a long term illness like this can be compared to other examples of great and testing times, like being at war for example, and should be looked at the same way.

We all learn through experiences like this and that confronting struggle can help strengthen us and teach us that that we can deal with a lot of seemingly less overwhelming things that life does throw our way.

The suffering brings families closer together and we rely on our friends and partners more as at day centres and sheltered projects. We come to live in the mental health system with other people who are also suffering and can be a source of strength for each other.

There is no need to panic once we are diagnosed with this terrifying illness and there are many forms of social and medical support on offer here as I have described this at various points above.

This of course is only true to the extent that the suffering does not make us want to commit suicide and I have to confess I still think about this from time to time when the symptoms are at the worst.

So I guess if there is a message here for people with schizophrenia it is that sometimes after lengthy struggles life is still worth it despite the fact we suffer. Getting over the worst times can be done but sadly this is not always the case and some people with schizophrenia do take their own lives.

These cases of suffering need to be looked at closely and is a difficult subject to cover which makes it far beyond the reaches of this book on anxiety.

Once the anxiety does subside however I am able to come round and appreciate the other profound influences in life like friends and family. This makes me able to lighten the mood that might have resulted in depression and prevents the illness dominating my life.

During the good phases I bounce back and that too is a powerful coping mechanism. The illness is not never ending and mood wise the good periods make up for the bad and sometimes but not always I know that the difficult phases will end another upturn is round the corner. Sadly again this will not be true for everybody.